AF443460

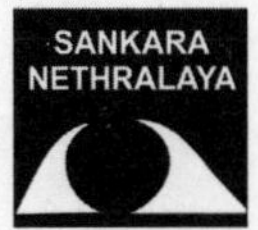

Sankara Nethralaya
Clinical Practice Patterns in
OPHTHALMOLOGY

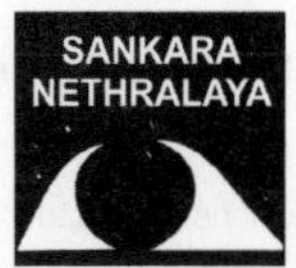

Sankara Nethralaya
Clinical Practice Patterns in
OPHTHALMOLOGY

Second Edition

Editor

SS Badrinath FRCS (Ed) (Hon. Causa)
President and Chairman Emeritus
Medical Research Foundation
Member of Board
Vision Research Foundation
Sankara Nethralaya
Chennai, Tamil Nadu, India

Co-editor

Prema Padmanabhan MS (Ophthalmology)
Medical Director and Director
Department of Cornea and Refractive Surgery
Medical Research Foundation
Sankara Nethralaya
Chennai, Tamil Nadu, India

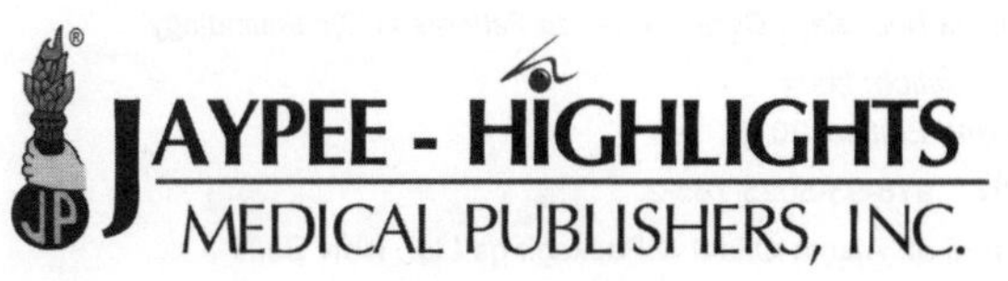

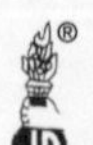

Jaypee Brothers Medical Publishers (P) Ltd.

Headquarters

Jaypee Brothers Medical Publishers (P) Ltd.
4838/24, Ansari Road, Daryaganj
New Delhi 110 002, India
Phone: +91-11-43574357
Fax: +91-11-43574314
Email: jaypee@jaypeebrothers.com

Overseas Offices

J.P. Medical Ltd.
83 Victoria Street, London
SW1H 0HW (UK)
Phone: +44-2031708910
Fax: +02-03-0086180
Email: info@jpmedpub.com

Jaypee-Highlights Medical Publishers Inc.
City of Knowledge, Bld. 237, Clayton
Panama City, Panama
Phone: +507-301-0496
Fax: +507-301-0499
Email: cservice@jphmedical.com

Jaypee Brothers Medical Publishers (P) Ltd.
17/1-B Babar Road, Block-B, Shaymali
Mohammadpur, Dhaka-1207, Bangladesh
Mobile: +08801912003485
Email: jaypeedhaka@gmail.com

Jaypee Brothers Medical Publishers (P) Ltd.
Shorakhute, Kathmandu, Nepal
Phone: +00977-9841528578
Email: jaypee.nepal@gmail.com

Website: www.jaypeebrothers.com
Website: www.jaypeedigital.com

Sankara Nethralaya Clinical Practice Patterns in Ophthalmology

First Edition: 2004
Second Edition: **2013**
ISBN : 978-93-5025-785-2
Printed at: Ajanta Offset & Packagings Ltd., New Delhi

To

Patients and physicians we dedicate,
this ophthalmic clinical consolidate
presenting a paper back of practices preferred
A few ancient revered, many modern adhered
compiled to make eye care uniform
so that, quality control becomes a norm

Preface to the Second Edition

The ever-increasing stockpile of scientific knowledge and our never-waning determination to keep pace with it, have been the compelling reasons for bringing out the second edition of the *Sankara Nethralaya Clinical Practice Patterns in Ophthalmology*.

The guiding philosophy remains the same—the use of technology to aid (without replacing) clinical judgment and an evidence-based treatment adapted to the Indian context. We have chosen to retain the step-by-step format in summarizing our approach to the management of commonly encountered diseases. This, we believe, is what makes this a ready-to-use clinical companion.

A few chapters have been added and some old ones modified wherever needed. Newer diagnostic tools, which have been found useful, have been included, and new treatment modalities described.

The popularity of the earlier edition of the book is, in itself, a tribute to the consultants of Sankara Nethralaya, Chennai, Tamil Nadu, India and has been the impetus for their renewed collective drive to make this a richer and more updated repository of their clinical wisdom.

We believe, this handbook in style and content, fulfills the need of practicing ophthalmologists who may not have the time or access to books and journals, but who believe in giving their patients the best of treatment. We hope, they will reach out for the book with the same enthusiasm as that with which it has been compiled.

SS Badrinath
Prema Padmanabhan

Preface to the First Edition

Let the word Sankara of Sankara Nethralaya ever remind me and my associates, His Holiness' command that there be missionary spirit in the project. Let the word Nethralaya constantly remind me and my colleagues that the place of our work is an alaya. Work will be our worship which we shall do with sincerity, dedication and utmost love.

Ever since this sacred pledge was taken 25 years ago, "Comprehensive Eye Care" has been the insignia of Sankara Nethralaya. In order to maintain the standards we have set for ourselves, we need to constantly update ourselves and upgrade our services to our patients. To ensure 'comprehensive care' in ophthalmology today, we often need to adopt a collaborative team approach and to maintain 'quality', we need to standardize that approach.

As the title suggests, this summarizes our approach at Sankara Nethralaya to the management of clinical entities commonly encountered in our ophthalmic practice. It is neither intended to be a formal textbook, nor it is meant to imply that other methods of treatment prescribed and practiced elsewhere are incorrect. The endeavor has been to create guidelines that are rational, practical and relevant to the Indian context. It combines the time-tested recipes of a 25-years clinical experience at Sankara Nethralaya with updated concepts of evolving thought processes all over the globe.

This compendium has been the result of a collective work of all the consultants of Sankara Nethralaya. On the occasion of the 25th anniversary of Sankara Nethralaya, we have great pleasure in sharing this with the ophthalmic community with the hope that it adds value and meaning to the quality of eye care rendered to our patients.

SS Badrinath

Prema Padmanabhan

Contents

Abbreviations

5-FU 5-fluorouracil
AC Anterior chamber
AC:A Accommodative convergence to accommodation ratio
ACG Acute angle-closure glaucoma
ACIOL Anterior chamber intraocular lens
AIDS Acquired immunodeficiency syndrome
AION Anterior ischemic optic neuropathy
AMT Amniotic membrane transplantation
ANA Antinuclear antibody
ANCA Antineutrophil cytoplasmic antibody
APMPPE Acute posterior multifocal placoid pigment epitheliopathy
APTT Activated partial thromboplastin time
ARC Abnormal retinal correspondence
ARMD Age-related macular degeneration
ARN Acute retinal necrosis
AVM Arteriovenous malformation
BCC Basal cell carcinoma
BCL Bandage contact lens
BCVA Best-corrected visual acuity
bd Twice daily
BHIB Brain heart infusion broth
BP Blood pressure
BRAO Branch retinal artery occlusion
BRVO Branch retinal vein occlusion
BSV Binocular single vision
BUT Break-up time (of tear film)
C/D Cup-disc ratio
CBC Complete blood count
CCT Central corneal thickness
CF Counting fingers
CHED Congenital hereditary endothelial dystrophy
CHRPE Congenital hypertrophy of retinal pigment epithelium
CIN Conjunctival intraepithelial neoplasia
CL Contact lens
CME Cystoid macular edema
CMV Cytomegalovirus
CN II Cranial nerve II (optic nerve)

CN III   Cranial nerve III (oculomotor nerve)
CN IV   Cranial nerve IV (trochlear nerve)
CN V   Cranial nerve V (trigeminal nerve)
CN VI   Cranial nerve VI (abducens nerve)
CN VII   Cranial nerve VII (facial nerve)
CNV   Choroidal neovascularization
CNVM   Choroidal neovascular membrane
CPEO   Chronic progressive external ophthalmoplegia
CRAO   Central retinal artery occlusion
CRP   C-reactive protein
CRVO   Central retinal vein occlusion
CSCR   Central serous chorioretinopathy
CSF   Cerebrospinal fluid
CSME   Clinically significant macular edema
CSNB   Congenital stationary night blindness
CSR   Central serous (chorio)retinopathy
CT   Computed tomography
CTC   Cyclopentolate-tropicamide-cyclopentolate
CVA   Cerebrovascular accident
CVS   Cardiovascular system
CWS   Cotton-wool spot
CXR   Chest X-ray
D   Diopter
DALK   Deep anterior lamellar keratoplasty
DC   Diopter cylinder
DCCT   Diabetes Control and Complication Trial
DCG   Dacryocystogram
DCR   Dacryocystorhinostomy
DD   Disc diameter
DLC   Differential leukocyte count
DLEK   Deep lamellar endothelial keratoplasty
DM   Diabetes mellitus
DNA   Deoxyribonucleic acid
DOV   Dimness of vision
DS   Diopter sphere
DSEK   Descemet's stripping endothelial keratoplasty
DVD   Dissociated vertical deviation
DVT   Deep venous thrombosis
EBV   Epstein–Barr virus
ECCE   Extracapsular cataract extraction
ECG   Electrocardiogram
EDTA   Ethylenediaminetetraacetic acid
EEG   Electroencephalogram
EIA   Enzyme immunosorbent
ELISA   Enzyme-linked immunosorbent assay

EMG	Electromyogram
ENT	Ear, nose, and throat specialist (otolaryngologist)
EOG	Electro-oculogram
EOM	Extraocular muscle
ERD	Exudative retinal detachment
ERG	Electroretinogram
ESR	Erythrocyte sedimentation rate
EUA	Examination under anesthesia
Fab	Fragment antigen-binding
FAZ	Foveal avascular zone
FB	Foreign body
FDA	Food and Drug Administration
FDP	Frequency doubling perimetry
FDT	Forced duction test
FFA	Fundus fluorescein angiography
FML	Fluorometholone
FNAB	Fine needle aspiration biopsy
FTA/ABS	Fluorescent treponemal antibody absorbed
FVL	Functional visual loss
GA	Glass appointment
GCA	Giant cell arteritis
GHPC	Geographic helicoid peripapillary choroidopathy
GI	Gastrointestinal system
GVHD	Graft-versus-host disease
H/O	History of
HA+T	Homatropine + tropicamide
HBsAg	Hepatitis B surface antigen
HIV	Human immunodeficiency virus
HLA	Human leukocyte antigen
HM	Hand movements
HPE	Histopathological examination
HPV	Human papilloma virus
HRCT	High-resolution computed tomography
HRT	Heidelberg retinal tomography
HSV	Herpes simplex virus
HVF	Humphrey visual field
HZO	Herpes zoster ophthalmicus
IM	Intramuscular
IV	Intravenous
ICCE	Intracapsular cataract extraction
ICE	Iridocorneal endothelial syndrome
ICG	Indocyanine green angiography
IDDM	Insulin dependant diabetes mellitus
IHD	Ischemic heart disease

ILM	Internal limiting membrane
INO	Internuclear ophthalmoplegia
IO	Inferior oblique
IOFB	Intraocular foreign body
IOL	Intraocular lens
IOP	Intraocular pressure
IPCV	Idiopathic polypoidal choroidal vasculopathy
IR	Inferior rectus
IRMA	Intraretinal microvascular abnormalities
I-S	Inferior superior dioptric asymmetry
ISCEV	International Society for Clinical Electrophysiology of Vision
IUSG	International Uveitis Study Group
JIA	Juvenile idiopathic arthritis
JRA	Juvenile rheumatoid arthritis
K value	Keratometry value
KCS	Keratoconjunctivitis sicca
KISA%	$(K) \times (I–S) \times (AST) \times (SRAX) \times 100$ topographic index for keratoconus
KOH	Potassium hydroxide
KP	Keratic precipitate
LASIK	Laser stromal *in situ* keratomileusis
LFT	Liver function tests
LP	Light perception
LPS	Levator palpebrae superioris
LR	Lateral rectus
LVA	Low vision aid
MEWDS	Multiple evanescent white dot syndrome
MG	Myasthenia gravis
MI	Myocardial infarction
MMC	Mitomycin C
MMG	Mucous membrane grafting
MR	Medial rectus
MRA	Magnetic resonance angiography
MRI	Magnetic resonance imaging
MRV	Magnetic resonance venography
MS	Multiple sclerosis
Nd-YAG	Neodymium-yttrium-aluminum-garnet laser
NF-1, 2	Neurofibromatosis types 1 and 2
NFL	Nerve fiber layer
NHL	Non-Hodgkin's lymphoma
NLD	Nasolacrimal duct
NPDR	Nonproliferative diabetic retinopathy
NPL	No perception of light
NPO	Nil per os (nothing by mouth)
NRR	Neuroretinal rim

NSAID Nonsteroidal anti-inflammatory drug
NTG Normal-tension glaucoma
NVA Neovascularization of the angle
NVD Neovascularization of the optic disc
NVE Neovascularization elsewhere
NVG Neovascular glaucoma
NVI Neovascularization of the iris
OCT Optical coherence tomography
OD Oculus dexter (right eye)
OHT Ocular hypertension
OKN Optokinetic nystagmus
ONH Optic nerve head
ONSD Optic nerve sheath decompression
OS Oculus sinister (left eye)
OU Both eyes
PACG Primary angle-closure glaucoma
PAM Pigmented acquired melanosis; potential acuity meter
PAN Polyarteritis nodosa; periodic alternating nystagmus
PAS Peripheral anterior synechiae; periodic acid–Schiff
PCIOL Posterior chamber intraocular lens
PCO Posterior capsular opacification
PCR Polymerase chain reaction
PCV Polypoidal choroidal vasculopathy
PDR Proliferative diabetic retinopathy
PDS Pigmentary dispersion syndrome
PDT Photodynamic therapy
PED Pigment epithelial defect; persistent epithelial defect
PERG Pattern electroretinogram
PFV Persistent fetal vasculature
PHMB Polyhexamethylene biguanide
PHPV Persistent hyperplastic primary vitreous
PI Peripheral iridotomy
PIC Punctate inner choroidopathy
PK Penetrating keratoplasty
PMD Pellucid marginal degeneration
PMMA Polymethyl methacrylate
POAG Primary open-angle glaucoma
POHS Presumed ocular histoplasmosis syndrome
PORN Progressive outer retinal necrosis
PPBS Postprandial blood sugar
PPDR Preproliferative diabetic retinopathy
PPMD Posterior polymorphous corneal dystrophy

PPRF   Paramedian pontine reticular formation
PRN   Pro re nata
PRP   Panretinal photocoagulation
PTH   Parathyroid hormone
PTT   Prothrombin time
PVD   Posterior vitreous detachment
PVR   Proliferative vitreoretinopathy
PXF   Pseudoexfoliation syndrome
RA   Rheumatoid arthritis
RAPD   Relative afferent pupillary defect
Rb   Retinoblastoma
RD   Retinal detachment
RF   Rhematoid factor
RGP   Rigid gas permeable (of contact lenses)
Rh   Rhesus
RK   Refractive keratectomy
RNFL   Retinal nerve fiber layer
ROP   Retinopathy of prematurity
ROPLAS   Regurgitation on pressure over lacrimal sac
RP   Retinitis pigmentosa
RPE   Retinal pigment epithelium
RPR   Rapid plasma reagin
RRD   Rhegmatogenous retinal detachment
SACE   Serum angiotensin-converting enzyme
SCC   Squamous cell carcinoma
sec   Second(s)
SF   Short-term fluctuation
Si   Silicone (of oil)
SINS   Surgery-induced necrotizing scleritis
SITA   Swedish interactive threshold algorithm
SLE   Systemic lupus erythematosus
SLP   Scanning laser polarimetry
SLT   Selective laser trabeculoplasty
SO   Superior oblique
SOOF   Suborbicularis oculi fat pad
SMAS   Superficial mascular aponeurotic system
SPK   Superficial punctuate keratitis
SR   Superior rectus
SRAX   Skewed radial axis index
SRF   Subretinal fluid
SRNVM   Subretinal neovascular membrane
STD   Sexually transmitted disease
SUN   Standardization of Uveitis Nomenclature
(group)
TB   Tuberculosis
TED   Thyroid eye disease

TFT	Thyroid function tests
TG	Triglyceride
TIA	Transient ischemic attack
TLC	Total leukocyte count
TM	Trabecular meshwork
TNF	Tumor necrosis factor
tPA	Tissue plasminogen activator
TPHA	*Treponema pallidum* hemagglutination assay
TRD	Tractional retinal detachment
TSH	Thyroid stimulating hormone
TT	Tetenus toxoid
TTT	Transpupillary thermotherapy
UA	Urinalysis
UBM	Ultrasound biomicroscopy
URI	Upper respiratory infection
URTI	Upper respiratory tract infection
USG	Ultrasound
V 1, 2, 3	Ophthalmic, maxillary, and mandibular divisions of CN V
VA	Visual acuity
VDRL	Venereal disease research laboratory test
VEGF	Vascular endothelial growth factor
VEP	Visually evoked potential
VKC	Vernal keratoconjunctivitis
VKH	Vogt–Koyanagi–Harada syndrome
WBC	White blood cells
WHO	World Health Organization

1

Orbit and Oculoplasty

- Preoperative Evaluation
- Evaluation and Management of Ptosis
- Entropion
- Ectropion
- Trichiasis (Misdirected Lashes)
- Lid Lesions (Benign/Malignant Growth)
- Biopsy for Lid Pathologies
- Eyelid and Adnexal Injuries
- Thyroid Associated Ophthalmopathy
- Orbital Injuries including Fractures
- Orbital Fine Needle Aspiration Biopsy
- Indications for Computed Tomography
- Indications for Magnetic Resonance Imaging
- Dacryocystitis
- Dacryocystography
- Endoscopy
- Socket Evaluation
- Ocular Prosthesis
- Aesthetic Clinic

PREOPERATIVE EVALUATION

Preoperative preparation of the patient is as important to the success of a plastic procedure as the actual technique.

EVALUATION IN THE OCULOPLASTY DEPARTMENT

Patient Assessment-Psychological Implications

- The evaluation of a patient starts from the moment the patient steps into the consultation room till the entire course of his treatment.
- The purpose is to determine if plastic surgery is appropriate for a particular patient at a particular time.
- The motives, expectations and personality of the patient are to be assessed by observation and casual open-ended dialogue.
- Give the patient an information pamphlet on plastic surgery procedures outlining realistic expectations, preoperative and postoperative condition and possible side effects.
- Explain the available modalities of treatment for the particular condition with the risks and benefits of each.
- Explain the surgical procedure and the complications which are likely to occur, if the surgery is to be done under local or general anesthesia.
- Explain the realistic outcome of the surgery to the patient.
- Explain the need for multiple procedures or a staged treatment plan in the case of a complicated condition and the reasons if any particular surgery is contraindicated.
- Explain the need for taking grafts if required, the donor sites, the cosmetic implications, the post-

operative care of the donor site as well as the primary surgical site.

- Establishment of a positive relationship with the patient will pay well in the entire course of treatment of the patient.

MEDICOLEGAL IMPLICATIONS

Informed Consent

The modern standard of care requires the physician to inform the patient of the nature of the proposed treatment, alternate therapies including none, risks and reasonably expected benefits of each one and only then secure their consent.

Few Simple Rules

- Be kind to the patient
- Keep good records—essential for defense and is the best available evidence
- Inform the patient of all the possibilities and ask if he understood the same
- Never hesitate to get a second opinion if required
- Photographic documentation is essential.

GENERAL PHYSICAL EXAMINATION

- History of diabetes, hypertension, cardiovascular disorders, bronchial asthma
- History of respiratory tract infections—upper and lower
- History of bleeding diathesis
- History of seizures
- History of renal disorders—preoperative antibiotics, anesthetic medications
- History of allergies, sensitivities to any drugs
- Treatment history—intake of antiplatelet drugs, anticoagulants, etc.
- Family history of bleeding disorders, atopy.

In Case of a Child

- History of being born of a consanguinous marriage
- History of pregnancy-related complications—infections, drug intake
- *History of mode of delivery:*
  - Forceps delivery
  - Prolonged labor
- History of postnatal complications, milestones, vaccination, feeding habits.

INVESTIGATIONS

- *Baseline blood investigations:*
  - Hematocrit, TLC, DLC
  - Blood sugar
  - ESR
  - Bleeding time, clotting time, prothrombin time, partial thromboplastin time
  - Blood grouping and Rh typing
  - Crossmatching in cases where blood loss is expected
- Serum urea, creatinine
- Urinalysis, serologic tests and electrolyte studies based on any supporting clinical signs
- HIV, HBsAg, Hepatitis C
- Chest X-ray
- Baseline ECG a must in all patients above age of 40 years and echocardiogram if required
- Rule out foci of infection—regional and distant
- Ultrasonogram of the orbits
- CT scan of the orbits, brain/MRI in necessary cases
- Thyroid function tests—Free T3, T4, TSH, anti-thyroid antibodies
- Metastatic work-up in case of suspected metastases to the orbit:
  - CXR, CT scan chest
  - USG abdomen
  - X-ray long bones, bone scan
  - CT scan brain
  - Liver and renal function tests.

The Day Before Surgery

Anesthetist review: To explain the mode of anesthesia, proper premedication to be given, cardiovascular and respiratory assessment.

Surgeon's Review

- Check for good preoperative photographs
- Check for enucleation/evisceration/orbitotomy consent
- Explaining about the procedure
  - Removal of the eyeball or its contents respectively which would mean total loss of vision in the operated site
  - Orbitotomy—impairment of vision, limitation of ocular motility, double vision, lid droop, squinting can occur
- Check the donor graft site—hygiene and asepsis (Antiseptic mouthwash to be given in cases where buccal mucosal graft is planned).

On the Day of Surgery

- Monitoring of blood sugar, blood pressure
- Premedication, antibiotics, preparation of the patient.

Inside the Operation Theater

- The surgeon should speak to the patient and make him relaxed before starting the surgery
- Check the consent form
- Check and cross-check the eye undergoing the surgery
- Check the mode of anesthesia local/general anesthesia
- Check the anesthetic drug if local anesthesia is planned expiry date, contamination if any
- Check if the blood is ready as required
- Check if X-ray lobby is ready

- Check the availability of headlights, microscope, magnifying loupes
- Pathology department to be informed prior if frozen section is planned, things to be kept ready for imprint cytology
- Check the availability of the instruments required for surgery and their sterilization, review the suture materials
- Check the emergency department
- Combination of preoperative photographs and CT/ MRI scans, measurements should be in the operating room visible to the surgeon
- Markings on the skin should be done prior to distorting the tissues by injection and without pull on these tissues by the head drapes.

EVALUATION AND MANAGEMENT OF PTOSIS

HISTORY

- *Age of presentation:* Since birth/Acquired later in life
- Precipitating factor
- *Progression of the symptoms:*
  - Worsening
  - Duration of stable ptosis
  - Diurnal variation
  - Presence of other neurological problems
- History of trauma
- History of any eyelid/ocular surgery
- History of double vision
- Review of old photographs, if available.

EXAMINATION OF PTOSIS

- Facial asymmetry/dysmorphia
- Abnormal head posture (AHP)
- Periocular skin-scarring, mass lesions, dermato-chalasis
- Visual acuity
- Refraction
- Hirschberg/cover test
- Extraocular motility (EOM)
- Pupillary evaluation
- Slit-lamp evaluation—giant papillary conjunctivitis
- Fundus
- *Measurements:*
  - Palpebral fissure height (PFH)
  - Margin reflex distance (MRD 1 and 2)
  - Levator action (LPS)
  - Margin crease distance (MCD)
- Lid lag
- Lagophthalmos

- Bell's phenomenon
- Marcus Gunn jaw winking/other synkinetic movements
- Drooping of contralateral lid on manual ptosis correction
- Fatiguability/Cogan lid twitch
- Corneal sensation
- *Ancilliary tests:*
  - Phenylephrine test
  - Schirmer's test
  - Ice test.

NB: It is important to eliminate frontalis overaction while taking ptosis measurements:

1. Photographic documentation is a must showing the close-up of face with and without face turn or chin elevation in straight gaze—preferably postoperative and follow-up pictures with the same background.
2. Parent/patient counseling especially to explain postoperative problems of lid lag and lagophthalmos, possible complications and need for revision procedures.

SURGICAL APPROACH

Congenital Ptosis

- Early surgery is indicated if the ptosis is severe and the child is in the amblyogenic age group.
- If the visual axis is spared surgery is to be performed when the child is round 3 to 5 years old provided the child is cooperative for the initial assessment and subsequent follow-up.
- In the case of Marcus Gunn phenomenon with significant jaw wink.
  - LPS excision + Frontalis sling, early, if the child is within the amblyogenic age group and the ptosis is severe; preschool age if not.
- Mild and moderate ptosis with fair-to-good function of the LPS—plan for LPS resection

- Severe ptosis and/or poor LPS action—plan for frontalis sling
- *Bilateral ptosis:*
  - Same sitting if the ptosis is severe or symmetrical
  - Worse eye first if the ptosis is asymmetrical followed 6 months later by the fellow eye
- In cases of vertical squint, referral to squint surgeon to improve pseudoptosis.

Aponeurotic Ptosis

- Surgery is indicated for cosmetic or functional impairment
- Procedure of choice is external approach with LPS reinsertion/advancement under local anesthesia.

Neurogenic Ptosis

- Minimum 6 months of stable ptosis without further improvement is a must prior to surgery
- Correct the squint prior to the ptosis
- *Options:* Frontalis sling and occasionally LPS resection.

Myogenic Ptosis

- Tensilon test, neurologist referral in cases of suspected myogenic ptosis
- Crutch glasses can be prescribed in patients refusing surgery
- Frontalis sling with silicon rods with undercorrection may be considered.

Traumatic Ptosis

- Minimum 6 months stable period
- *Options include:* Exploration ± reinsertion of the LPS aponeurosis or frontalis sling
- Important to assess the adequacy of Bell's phenomenon and degree of extraocular muscle entrapment and restriction.

POSTOPERATIVE MANAGEMENT

- Look for epithelial defects (corneal status)
- Wound integrity
- Suture removal to be done on 5-7th postoperative day
- Assessment of the procedure objectively by measuring the palpebral fissure width
- Subjective assessment in terms of patient satisfaction
- Look for complications
- Final documentation with photographs to be made
- Cycloplegic refraction in case of children at GA
- Periodic annual evaluation is preferred.

REPEAT SURGERY

Overcorrection

Initial trial with lash traction/lid stretching. If not satisfactory by 3 to 6 weeks, then revision surgery. If overcorrection is causing exposure related problems, early release of sutures to be done.

Undercorrection

Repeat surgery after a minimum of 6 weeks. In case of persisting edema, preferable to wait until edema resolves.

ENTROPION

DEFINITION

It is the condition where there is an inturning of the upper or lower eyelid with posterior migration/ rounding of the posterior lid margin, eyelash contact against the cornea, etc. It may be partial or complete, intermittent or constant and symptomatic or asymptomatic.

EVALUATION

History

- *Symptoms (of present illness):*
  - Irritation, FB sensation, redness
  - Tearing
  - Discharge
  - Light sensitivity
  - Visual loss
  - Interference with overall functioning and quality of life
  - Duration (intermittent or constant)
  - Aggravating or relieving factors.
- *Past history:*
  - Chronic blepharoconjunctivitis
  - Glaucoma medications
  - Trachoma
  - Trauma/burns (thermal/chemical)
  - Ocular or eyelid surgery
  - Radiation
  - Stevens-Johnson's syndrome, ocular cicatricial pemphigoid, etc.
- *Medical history:*
  - Diabetes mellitus
  - Systemic hypertension
  - Bleeding diathesis
  - Aspirin/anticoagulant intake
  - Anesthetic complications.

- Surgical history
- Drug allergies.

EXAMINATION

- General condition
- Facies
- Involutional changes of face—brows, upper eyelids, lower eyelids, dermatochalasis
- Complete ophthalmic evaluation—with specific emphasis on corneal examination—corneal epithelium, sensation, scarring, tear film, etc.
- *Upper eyelid entropion:*
  - Brow position
  - Vertical palpebral aperture
  - Margin reflex distance 1
  - Levator function
  - Superior lid crease
  - Lash position and direction
  - Posterior lid margin
  - Meibomian gland orifices—position, inspissation, distichiasis
  - Tarsal conjunctiva—shortening, scarring, integrity, thickening
  - Spontaneous eversion—floppy eyelid
- *Lower eyelid:*
  - Position
  - Lid margin including retraction
  - Lash position and direction
  - Horizontal lid laxity—distraction test, snap back test
  - Medial canthal tendon integrity
  - Punctal position and patency
  - Capsulopalpebral fascia integrity
  - Conjunctival scarring
  - Dermatochalasis
  - Suborbicularis oculi fat/superficial musculo-aponeurotic system (SOOF/SMAS) descent
  - Precipitation on forced eyelid closure.

- *Oral examination:*
  - Labial mucosa
  - Buccal mucosa
  - Hard palate mucosa
  - Dental/gingival hygiene

INVESTIGATIONS

- Tests for general fitness for surgery/anesthesia
- Coagulation tests
- Photographic documentation.

MANAGEMENT

- Educate, counsel patient
- Informed consent
- Temporary procedures (lower eyelid)—taping, Botox injection, Quickert's sutures, etc.
- Definitive surgery—lid tightening, eyelid retractor plication/reinsertion, margin rotation/tarsal fracture, spacer graft with MMG, etc.
- Consider blepharoplasty when necessary.

ECTROPION

DEFINITION

It is the condition where there is an outward turning of the upper or lower eyelid with anterior migration/ rounding of the posterior lid margin, ectropion of the puncta, keratinization of the conjunctiva and shortening of the anterior lamella of the eyelid. It may be partial or complete, symptomatic or asymptomatic.

EVALUATION

History

- *Symptoms (of present illness):*
  - Tearing
  - Irritation, redness
  - Discharge
  - Visual loss—intermittent blurring, permanent deficit
  - Interference with overall functioning and quality of life
  - Duration (intermittent or constant)
  - Aggravating or relieving factors.
- *Past history:*
  - Chronic blepharoconjunctivitis
  - Trauma
  - Ocular, eyelid or facial surgery
  - Radiation, burns (thermal/chemical).
- *Medical history:*
  - Cicatrizing dermatological conditions- ichthyosis, actinic keratosis, contact dermatitis
  - Diabetes mellitus
  - Systemic hypertension
  - Bleeding disorders
  - Aspirin/anticoagulant intake
  - Anesthetic complications
- Surgical history
- Drug allergies.

EXAMINATION

- General condition
- Facies
- Involutional changes of face—brows, upper eyelids, lower eyelids, dermatochalasis
- Complete ophthalmic evaluation with specific emphasis on corneal examination—corneal epithelium, sensation, scarring, tear film, etc.
- *Upper eyelid ectropion:*
  - Brow position
  - Vertical palpebral aperture
  - Margin reflex distance 1
  - Levator Function
  - Superior lid crease
  - Lash position and direction
  - Posterior lid margin, keratinization of conjunctiva
  - Meibomian gland orifices—position, inspissation, distichiasis
  - Tarsal conjunctiva—shortening, scarring, thickening
  - Spontaneous eversion—floppy eyelid
  - Scarring of the eyelid/eyebrow/forehead skin.
- *Lower eyelid:*
  - Position
  - Lid margin including retraction
  - Lash position and direction
  - Horizontal lid laxity—distraction test, snap back test
  - Medial canthal tendon integrity
  - Punctal position and patency
  - Capsulopalpebral fascia integrity
  - Conjunctival scarring
  - Steatoblepharon
  - Dermatochalasis
  - SOOF/SMAS descent
  - Evaluation of the lacrimal secretory and drainage function

- *Other:*
  - Upper lid dermatochalasis-ipsilateral/contra-lateral eye
  - Retroauricular skin
  - Supraclavicular skin
  - Inner arm skin
  - Skin of anterior/medial thigh.

INVESTIGATIONS

- Tests for general fitness for surgery/anesthesia
- Coagulation tests
- Photographic documentation.

MANAGEMENT INCLUDING PRINCIPLES

- Educate, counsel patient
- Dermatology consultation if indicated (Cicatricial ectropion)
- Informed consent
- Punctal eversion-punctal inversion sutures, punctoplasty
- Involutional laxity—horizontal lid tightening—lateral tarsal strip, block excision, lateral canthal sling, etc.
- Anterior lamellar cicatricial changes—scar release with full thickness skin graft
- Tarsal ectropion—lid retractor reinsertion, tarso-conjunctival resection
- Consider blepharoplasty at the same sitting.

TRICHIASIS (MISDIRECTED LASHES)

HISTORY

- Trachoma
- History of drug ingestion of fever (Stevens-Johnson syndrome)
- Trauma/Burns
- Past history of treatment

EXAMINATION

- Extent of misdirected lashes (diagrammatic representation is ideal)
- Lid position
- Vision
- Puncta
- Fornices (symblepharon)
- Conjunctival scarring
- Corneal status (staining—SPK, ulcer)

MANAGEMENT

- Manual epilation (especially if there are very few misdirected lashes)
- Argon laser epilation
- Electroepilation
- Cryotherapy—this may be combined with posterior lamellar advancement ± mucous membrane graft in cases with posterior lamellar shortening.

LID LESIONS
(BENIGN/MALIGNANT GROWTH)

HISTORY

- Duration
- Rate of growth, mode of onset (sudden/gradual), change of color, bleeding, ulceration
- Any previous operation or biopsy—details if available including histopathology slides and paraffin blocks for review by our Ocular Pathology Department
- Any swelling in the head and neck or elsewhere in the body
- Associated ocular disease
- Major systemic illness.

EXAMINATION

- Detailed description of the eyelid lesion as in a general surgery examination (surface, consistency, etc.)
- A simple diagrammatic description with measurements, arrows, etc.
- Examine for condition of other lid, skin, eyelid margin (entropion, ectropion), lagophthalmos
- Always evert the lids and examine the posterior surface
- Examine the bulbar and palpebral conjunctiva and corneal surface in detail
- Look for skin ulceration, blood-stained discharge, loss of cilia
- Examine for preauricular and cervical lymph nodes
- Examine the rest of the face, body where applicable
- Inspection of other body areas for donor sites for planned reconstructive procedure (e.g. retro-auricular area, oral cavity).

MANAGEMENT

- To be examined and managed by Oculoplasty Consultant
- Photographic documentation of all cases
- In case of extensive lesions with possibility of orbital spread, USG orbit, CT scan orbit as applicable must be asked for
- Histopathological examination (HPE) slide review, where available by Ocular Pathologist
- Clinical diagnosis of benign/malignant lid lesion to be made in all cases with a detailed plan for management including technique of reconstruction
- In a suspected chalazion, incision and curettege is done and the curetted material should be sent for HPE, especially, in cases of recurrent swelling and in an older patient
- In small lesions, excision biopsy to be performed
- In case of benign large lesions, excision biopsy with appropriate technique of eyelid reconstruction
- In case of suspected malignant lesions, excision under frozen section control (Ocular Pathologist to be given advance notice of the same) with appropriate reconstruction
- It is nearly always necessary to obtain tissue diagnosis prior to referral to Oncologist
- In large tumors, incisional biopsy/exenteration as appropriate (arrange for blood transfusion as applicable)
- In case of HPE diagnosis of a malignancy, appropriate referral to Oncologist with a case summary, copy of HPE reports and HPE slides or block as appropriate
- Postoperative documentation in all cases
- Video documentation (academic), where needed

FOLLOW-UP

- As appropriate
- Removal of sutures can be done in the OPD; general anesthesia may be needed for pediatric age group.

BIOPSY FOR LID PATHOLOGIES

Features suggestive of malignancy and the necessity for biopsy:
- *Lesions which:*
  - Bleed easily
  - Spontaneously ulcerate
  - Increase in size
  - Have localized loss of eye lashes
- Any inflammatory lesion which pursues a relentless course.
- Lesion which does not respond to the usual therapy.
- Any growing lid lesion/recurrent stye/chronic rodent ulcer
- *Lesion which has:*
  - Pearly telangiectatic changes in an area of cutaneous disturbance
  - An area of diffuse induration
  - A scirrhous retracted area
  - Loss of eyelid margin architecture
- Involvement of regional lymph nodes.

Choice of a biopsy technique is based on:
a. Location of the lesion
b. Suspected histological diagnosis
c. Should minimize cosmetic defect
d. Should interfere the least with further surgery

The varied biopsy techniques are:
a. Punch biopsy
b. Shave biopsy
c. Excision biopsy
d. Incision biopsy

The goal of biopsy: To remove tissue which is representative of the lesion.

The requisites are:
- The specimen should be of adequate size

- Should include some normal tissue for comparison
- The specimen should be deep enough to include the base of the lesion
- Use of sharp delicate instruments and gentle handling of tissue to prevent crushing artifacts
- Orient the pathologist to the area by marking it or by drawing a simple diagram or pin the specimen with stainless steel pins or hypodermic needles.

Punch Biopsy

- Gives a cylinder of tissue.
- Different sizes of the punches are available with a circular sharp cutting edge
- Sizes are varying from 2 to 8 mm
- Most commonly used is 3 or 4 mm size punch
- Unsuitable in globe and adnexal lesions because of close proximity to the globe.

Shave Biopsy

- Gives a disc of tissue
- Used for a lesion whose major component is protruding above the skin, i.e. only for superficial lesions; not for a melanoma.

Excision Biopsy

- Simultaneous biopsy and excision of a tumor
- The advantage is that it provides direct visualization and excellent tissue control
- For best cosmetic results make an elliptical incision which incorporates the lesion and 1 to 2 mm of normal tissue
- Mark the area initially, excise the skin ellipse with 15 blade, mark the temporal or nasal aspect of the lesion with suture followed by suturing the wound.

Incision Biopsy

- To get a small but sufficient amount of tissue for diagnosis
- An area of normal appearing tissue is also included

- The advantage is that it provides direct visualization and ensures adequate sample harvestation.

  In a patient with a suspicious lid lesion, determine if a biopsy is indicated and what type would be appropriate.

- A probable benign lesion which is cosmetically unacceptable—shave biopsy
- A benign large lesion—excision biopsy with appropriate technique of lid reconstruction
- A probable malignant lesion which is small—primary excision with lid reconstruction
- A probable malignant lesion which is large—an incision biopsy/a small trephine punch is ideal
- Large malignant lesions—surgical removal under frozen section (pathologist informed beforehand) + extensive lid reconstruction
- Malignant lesions with invasion of adjacent soft tissues—subtotal or total exenteration.

EYELID AND ADNEXAL INJURIES

HISTORY

- Details of mode of injury—exact detailed description to be obtained from patient, witnesses
- Possibility of foreign body to be explored by detailed history
- First aid, details of treatment taken earlier including Inj tetanus toxoid
- Any associated injuries—head injuries, fractures, etc. to be specifically asked for
- General condition—systemic disease.

EXAMINATION

- Use disposable gloves when examining the patient
- Evaluate the general condition of the patient and if sick or unstable, urgent evaluation by Physician/ Anesthetist/Consultant in the emergency
- If general condition is poor, a decision regarding shifting the patient out of Sankara Nethralaya and to an appropriate hospital may need to be taken urgently
- All injuries to be examined and described in detail; a simple diagrammatic representation is appropriate
- Remove any glass pieces, dirt or foreign material and clean the wound with saline/distilled water
- Evaluate pupils and rule out relative afferent pupillary defect (RAPD) in all cases
- In case of profuse bleeding, inform the trauma consultant urgently
- In all cases look for associated orbital injuries— hematoma, fractures
- Perform a complete ophthalmic examination in all cases and rule out associated globe injuries
- CT scan of the orbit and brain may need to be done in case skull or orbit fractures are suspected.

MANAGEMENT

- Inj. TT 0.5 ml intramascular (if not already given)
- Nil orally till further orders
- Physician/Anesthetist opinion for fitness as appropriate
- Trauma Consultant to be informed urgently
- Arrange repair/reconstruction in MOT
- Documentation of all cases is essential—to be done in Emergency/Ward/Operation theater
- Urgent repair/reconstruction of eyelid injuries to be combined with any globe repair if present. If no associated globe injuries, lid surgery to be scheduled within 24 hours
- Repair may necessitate specialized techniques, e.g. skin grafting in injuries with loss of tissue, eyelid burns. These may need to be arranged for
- Postoperative evaluation and documentation at regular intervals.

GUIDELINES FOR DETAILED EXAMINATION OF MASS LESIONS OF THE ORBIT

Comprehensive History

- Presenting complaint to be recorded in chronological order
- Details of presenting symptoms and associated history
- Progression of symptoms
- Precipitating factors/events, e.g. trauma, physical straining
- Past treatment if any
- Response to treatment if any
- Presence of any systemic mass lesions elsewhere
- Visual compromise in terms of acuity, diplopia, blunting of colors
- Personal history in terms of weight loss, appetite, smoking, exposure to pets
- History of exposure STD if indicated
- History of contact with TB.

Evaluation of a Case of Proptosis

- Visual acuity
- Refraction
- Color vision
- Pupils
- Extraocular Motility/Hirschberg/Cover test
- Intraocular pressure (IOP)
- Slit-lamp examination
- Fundus
- Facial asymmetry/dysmorphia
- Exophthalmometry (Hertel's/Nafziger)
- Globe displacement—horizontal and vertical (2 ruler test)
- *Eyelids:*
  - Position (retraction, inf. scleral show, lateral flare)
  - Margin-reflex distance (MRD1)
  - Palpebral fissure height (PFH)
  - Lagophthalmos
- *Palpation:*
  - Orbit
  - Thyroid
  - Regional lymph nodes
- Globe retropulsion (RBR)
- Pulsation/Thrill/Bruit
- Valsalva
- Cranial nerves examination (II, III, IV, V, VI)
- *Systemic:* Skin, oral and nasal examination
- *Imaging:* USG, CT, MRI.

6 Ps: *Pain, Proptosis, Progression, Palpation, Pulsation, Periorbital changes.*

Systemic Evaluation

- Look for any masses in the body
- Lymphadenopathy
- Organomegaly
- Evaluation by allied specialists.

Investigations

- To be tailored to the nature of the presenting complaints

- Special investigations in view of planned surgery done
- USG B-scan orbit
- CT scan orbit (if the previous CT does not correlate with the current clinical findings or is more than a year old)
- MRI to be reserved for specific situations only.

Surgical Approach

- Informed special consent to be obtained in all cases regarding the risk for visual loss
- Depending on the location of the tumor and the nature of the lesion medial, lateral, superior, inferior and anterior orbitotomy
- Preference to be given to excisional biopsy for potentially resectable tumors
- Incisional biopsy for extensive infiltrative lesions/ debulking of the tumor
- Frozen section to be reserved in special situations and lab to be informed in advance for the same
- Intraoperatively both eyes to be prepared to enable pupillary evaluation
- Six hours postoperative when patient is conscious and oriented, pupillary evaluation and gross visual acuity to be checked. Methylprednisolone may be indicated in certain cases
- Drain to be removed when flow is minimal to nil (2–3 days)
- Suture removal to be done on 6th to 7th day
- Depending on biopsy report further line of management in terms of chemotherapy/radiotherapy/ follow-up is to be planned.

FOLLOW-UP

- At each visit, documentation of wound integrity, pupillary reaction, extra-ocular movement (EOM), Diplopia if any, visual acuity and Hertel's at six weeks postoperative
- If residual mass lesion is present, follow-up frequency tailored according to type of the lesion, including evaluation by allied specialists.

THYROID ASSOCIATED OPHTHALMOPATHY

DEFINITION

It is the condition where the eyeball and ocular adnexal structures (eyelid, extraocular muscles, orbital fat and optic nerve) are variably affected resulting in functional and cosmetic derangement of the patient related to autoimmune disease of the thyroid gland, sometimes with dysfunction of the thyroid gland.

EVALUATION

History

Ophthalmic

- Prominence of the eyes
- Wide eyed appearance
- Redness, irritation, tearing
- Blurred vision, blunting of colors
- Double vision
- Inability to close eyes
- Are the symptoms present in one or both eyes, intermittent or persistent, duration. Impact on daily quality of life.

Systemic

- Previous history of thyroid disease—hyper/hypo/euthyroid, thyroid swelling, surgery, radioactive or medical treatment, etc.
- Weight loss, palpitation, heat intolerance, dysmenorrhea/menorrhagia, altered bowel habits, increased appetite, etc.
- Diabetes mellitus—age of onset and nature of control
- Severe anemia (Pernicious), vitiligo, other autoimmune disorders
- Systemic hypertension
- History of smoking—duration, frequency.

Examination

See attached ITEDS/VISA forms.

Management Principles

- Determine above parameters
- Identify parameters for urgent/immediate intervention
  - Exposure keratopathy, optic neuropathy
- Appropriate investigations
  - Perimetry, Ultrasound study of the orbit, CT/ MRI scan of the orbit
- Educate and counsel patient regarding natural course of disease including need for frequent follow-up and warning symptoms of visual compromise.

To Stop Smoking

- Endocrinology referral and systemic management as indicated
- Supportive therapy—lubricants, taping, punctual occlusion, moisture goggles, prisms in spectacles
- Surgical
  - Acute—tarsorrhaphy/canthotomy/cantholysis, Orbital decompression
  - Residual disease
    - Severe disfiguring proptosis—Orbital decompression
    - Strabismus—strabismus surgery
    - Eyelid retraction—lid retraction repair +/- blepharoplasty
- Ongoing ophthalmic and general medical care.

ORBITAL INJURIES INCLUDING FRACTURES

HISTORY

- Details of mode of injury—exact detailed description to be obtained from patient, witnesses
- Possibility of foreign bodies (FBs) to be explored by detailed history
- First aid, details of treatment taken earlier including Inj. Tetanus toxoid
- Any associated injuries—head injuries, fractures, etc. to be specifically asked for
- General condition—systemic disease
- History of double vision, numbness or abnormal sensations over lower lid, cheek, or upper lid of affected side to be asked for
- Difficulty in opening mouth, chewing, etc.

EXAMINATION

- Use disposable gloves when examining the patient
- Evaluate the general condition of the patient and if sick or unstable, urgent evaluation by Physician/Anesthetist/Consultant in the Emergency
- If general condition is poor, a decision regarding shifting the patient out of Sankara Nethralaya and to an appropriate hospital may need to be taken urgently
- All injuries to be examined and described in detail; a simple diagrammatic representation is appropriate
- Rule out globe injury
- Remove any glass pieces, dirt or foreign material and clean the wound with saline/distilled water
- In case of profuse bleeding, inform the Oculoplasty/Trauma Consultant urgently
- Evaluate pupils and rule out RAPD in all cases
- In case of profuse bleeding, inform the Oculoplasty/Trauma Consultant urgently

- Look for and rule out proptosis/enophthalmos
- Rule out subcutaneous emphysema by looking for crepitus
- Gently palpate the orbital margins and facial bones for any point tenderness, irregularity or deformity
- Evaluate ocular motility and look for double vision
- Document double vision with Hess and diplopia charting whenever possible
- Perform Hertel's exophthalmometry whenever required and possible
- Rule out infraorbital nerve hypoesthesia.

MANAGEMENT

- Photographic documentation of all cases
- In case of proptosis, lubricant therapy, taping as applicable to prevent corneal exposure
- Ultrasound examination of orbit to rule out hematoma, etc. when needed
- X-ray orbits, CT scan orbit with axial and coronal cuts for documentation and to rule out fractures
- Oral antibiotics, NSAIDs, etc. as appropriate
- Use of icepacks in the early stages postinjury to reduce swelling, pain
- Inj. TT 0.5 ml intramascular if not already given
- Inform Trauma/Oculoplasty Consultant
- Advise patient not to blow the nose, especially if fracture of the medial orbital wall is suspected
- Conservative/surgical treatment on basis of extent of fractures, symptoms and signs. Surgical repair usually after 10 to 14 days
- Serial Hess and diplopia charting to evaluate progress
- Referral to Faciomaxillary Surgeon or Neurosurgeon when appropriate.

ORBITAL FINE NEEDLE ASPIRATION BIOPSY

INDICATIONS

- In tumors where histological confirmation is needed but primary treatment will not be surgical
- Identification of unresectable orbital tumors especially epithelial lesions
- Deep orbital lesion where surgery is risky with technical difficulty
- Diagnosis of cavernous sinus syndrome lesions which enter the orbit
- Metastatic tumors to the orbit
- Optic nerve lesions are biopsied only when vision has progressed to blindness or near blindness
- CT scan suggestive of lacrimal fossa malignancy or lymphoid lesions can be biopsied
- Orbital abscesses
- Aspiration of hematoma
- Suspected antibiomas and pseudotumor
- Debilitated or aged patients who are at risk for anesthesia or surgery.

PRE-REQUISITES

- Availability of an expert Cytopathologist
- Patient selection—fine needle aspiration biopsy (FNAB) gives only a small sample. Hence it is not as useful in patients for whom the differential diagnosis includes a choice between a benign and malignant tumor with similar microscopic features
- Anticipate the potential complications. Hence, it should not be done if it will not affect the choice of treatment
- The results are useful only if a positive result is obtained. False negative diagnoses also do occur because of sampling errors/fibrous tissue/ carcinomas with large fibrous component or prominent inflammatory component

- CT and ultrasound be done prior to FNAB for tumor location, dimensions and relationship to the ocular structures
- GA clearance for pediatric cases.

TECHNIQUE

- Explain the procedure, implications, necessity for further surgery if FNAB is not diagnostic or gives a confusing picture
- Ultrasound B-scan to locate the orbital mass and to guide the needle
- Anesthesia is usually not required in adults but in children general anesthesia is required
- A 3.75 cm/22 G Needle is taken on a 20 cc syringe mounted in a pistol grip holder. A one inch needle is used in children
- Under ultrasound guidance one enters the orbit through the upper or lower lid in the appropriate quadrant. Avoid direct entry over or under the globe
- No aspiration pressure is applied till the tumor is entered
- Once the mass is entered negative suction is applied as the needle is advanced and retracted slightly with small changes in angulation within the tumor
- Negative suction is released before the needle is withdrawn
- Immediately prepare the specimen by fixing it in 95 percent alcohol or immediately transfer the contents into a test tube containing heparin solution for cytospin
- Residual tissue in the needle if fixed in 4 percent formaldehyde and kept for cell block preparation and staining
- Pressure patch is applied for an hour or longer if necessary.

COMPLICATIONS

- Retrobulbar hemorrhage
- Globe perforation
- Vision loss

- Metastatic tumor seeding along the needle tract—very rare
- Ptosis
- Motility disturbances.

CONTRAINDICATIONS

- Vascular tumors such as arteriovenous malformations, orbital varices and hemangiomas
- Dermoids—leakage of cyst contents gives rise to intense inflammatory reaction
- Benign lacrimal gland tumors are not usually biopsied.

CT SCAN GUIDED ORBITAL FINE NEEDLE ASPIRATION BIOPSY

Indications

- For small lesions and posteriorly located lesions
- In deeply located lesions where ultrasound cannot image
- Lesions in the muscle cone especially optic nerve lesions in eyes which are nearly blind/are blind.

Technique

For Small and Posterior Lesions

- Needle is inserted first unattached to the syringe and pistol grip while positioning the patient in the scanner
- Check the location of the tip with scanner. If misplaced, reposition till it is within the mass
- Then attach the syringe with the pistol grip and do the aspiration.

For Optic Nerve Lesions

- Enter laterally through the lower lid and direct the needle up and medially
- Engage the optic nerve with the needle with a characteristic feel and the globe retracts slightly. The globe moves with the needle movement
- Evaluate the position and do the aspiration.

INDICATIONS FOR COMPUTED TOMOGRAPHY

- Proptosis
- Suspected orbital mass—location, size, shape, involved structures, density, calcification, contrast enhancement, bony change
- Unexplained optic neuropathy, visual field abnormalities, disc edema—contrast enhanced computed tomography (CT) of brain and orbits gives a picture of chiasma and retrochiasmal pathways for intracranial masses
- Orbital and ocular trauma—orbital and nasoethmoidal fractures, intraorbital soft tissue trauma, intraocular or orbital foreign body.
- Motility disorders—combined CT brain and orbits helps to localize lesions in cerebral cortex, brainstem, cerebellum, cranial nerves or extraocular muscles
- Orbital inflammation or infection—specific signs help in delineation like multiple muscle enlargement of Grave's ophthalmopathy, diffuse or localized orbital soft tissue enhancement in pseudotumor, cellulitis with subperiosteal abscess and sinusitis
- Pretreatment planning for radiotherapy
- Preoperative planning for craniofacial reconstructive surgery
- Pre-MR imaging evaluation to rule out orbital or ocular metallic foreign body (in certain selected areas)
- Bony or ossifying lesions of the orbit.

THREE DIMENSIONAL CT

It uses volume-based computerized reconstructions of thin axial sections—1.5 mm slices or contour surface imaging.

Indications

- In neurosurgery and craniofacial reconstructions especially in craniosynostosis and congenital

craniofacial deformities—preoperative three dimensional viewing of bony anatomy, orbital morphology and volume, globe position, soft tissue volumes
- To create orbitocranial prostheses which are used as models for tissue excision, as bone graft templates, as alloplastic implants
- To evaluate post-traumatic enophthalmos after orbital fractures due to the accuracy of volume measurement with 3D-CT
- Evaluation and management of orbital tumors—for evaluation of orbital osteomas, for detection of residual orbital neurofibroma, for reconstructive planning after extensive resection of orbitocranial malignant teratomas.

Advantages of CT

- Excellent anatomical definition of bony and soft tissue anatomy
- Cheaper and affordable than MRI
- Good spatial resolution
- Less sensitivity to patient motion—motion artifacts are lessened.

Disadvantages of CT

- Radiation exposure approximately 2 to 3 rads
- Allergic reactions to iodinated contrast dye
- Poor contrast between some adjacent soft tissues which are isodense
- Artifacts are produced by dense bone and metallic objects
- Sagittal imaging is not possible.
- Not indicated in pregnancy.

Disadvantages of Three Dimensional CT

- Time investment for each study
- Cost
- Absolute necessity of strictly limiting patient movement
- Increased radiation exposure with multiple thin slices.

INDICATIONS FOR MAGNETIC RESONANCE IMAGING

INDICATIONS

- Identification, localization and delineation of soft tissue lesions
- Optic canal lesions and lesions around optic canal, to identify intracranial extension
- Mass lesion surrounding the optic nerve.

ADVANTAGES

- Can be done in pregnancy
- Greater image resolution of central nervous system (CNS) and other soft tissues which are isodense on CT
- Better detection of subtle pathologic changes
- Less artifacts from metallic objects, dense bone, dental fill-ups
- Allows imaging in multiple planes without patient repositioning or image reformatting
- No risk of ionizing radiation
- Better delineation of soft tissues in crowded bony regions as posterior fossa, optic canal, orbital apex due to less bony interference
- Better for evaluation of intracranial extension of intraorbital lesions
- Reveals excellent contrast between orbital fat, extraocular muscles and intraconal structures.

CONTRAINDICATIONS

- Absolute—presence of ferromagnetic cerebral aneurysmal clips or cardiac pacemakers
- *Relative:*
  - Iron foreign body in the eye or orbit
  - Claustrophobia

- Metallic prosthetic heart valves
- Uncooperative patient.

DISADVANTAGES

- Higher cost of equipment and site preparation
- Slower scanning times
- Greater sensitivity to movement artifact
- Poorer imaging of bony structures
- Poor spatial resolution—spatial blurring due to intense bright signals from orbital fat in T1 images degrades image quality.

DACRYOCYSTITIS

CONGENITAL DACRYOSTENOSIS
History

- Age of onset
- Duration and severity of symptoms
- Unilateral/bilateral
- History of watering/wet looking eyes
- History of discharge and matting of lashes
- History of symptoms worsening with respiratory infection
- History of application of eyedrops
- History of massage and the technique
- Details of any procedure done under anesthesia—probing
- History of redness and swelling of the eyes
- History of prematurity
- History of trauma.

Clinical Examination

- Mucoid/mucopurulent discharge in the medial canthal area
- Dried mucoid discharge on the lashes
- Increased tear meniscus
- Skin maceration
- Fixation and following of light
- Corneal status
- Digital tension
- Extraocular movements
- Fundus examination.

Examination in the Oculoplasty Department

- Position of lids
- Examination of puncta
- Surface abnormalities
- Medial canthal mass
- Lacrimal—cutaneous fistula
- ROPLAS sign—regurgitation on pressure over lacrimal sac region
- Anterior segment examination.

Management

The nature and course of the condition to be discussed in detail with the parents.

Conservative Treatment

- Lid hygiene
- Antibiotics - vanmycetin eyedrops 4 times/day x 2 weeks
- *Massage - Crigler's technique:*
    - 20 strokes every time 3 times a day
    - Correct procedure is explained to the parents

This is done for two months up to the age of 6 months. If this fails probing and syringing is done.

Probing and Syringing of Lacrimal System

- Ideal time is 6 to 9 months of age
- General anesthesia with intubation is necessary
- After punctal dilatation, Bowman's probe of adequate size is passed through puncta and maneuvered through the lacrimal system to reach the floor of the nose
- Type of resistance (hard or membranous) and approximate level of the block/site of give-way is noted
- Nasal endoscope is used to visualize probe in inferior meatus
- Inferior turbinate infracture/intubation is done if needed
- Syringing is done to confirm patency of the lacrimal system
- Nature, site and percentage of regurtation, if present, is noted
- Continue topical antibiotics and massage for 2 to 3 months
- If this fails, probing is repeated after 3 months.

Persistence of Symptoms and Bony Block

- Periodic follow-up is essential
- Dacryocystorhinostomy at the age of 5 years or earlier if situation demands.

ACUTE DACRYOCYSTITIS

History

- History of watering and discharge—duration and severity
- History of pain, redness, swelling in the medial part of the eye
- History of fever
- History of previous episodes
- History of any treatment taken
- History of sinusitis, nasal blockage.

Clinical Examination

- Swelling, edema and erythema in the lacrimal sac region below the medial canthal region
- Warmth and tenderness of lacrimal sac region
- Tear stasis
- Fistula formation
- Visual functions-visual acuity
- Pupillary reactions
- Ocular motility evaluation.

Examination in the Oculoplasty Department

- Examination of lids and puncta
- Preseptal or orbital cellulitis
- Evaluation of proptosis, if present.

Guidelines in the Management

- Avoid probing and irrigation of canalicular system till infection subsides
- Warm compresses
- Topical antibiotics of limited value when stasis is there
- Oral antibiotics of value in mild-to-moderate cases
- Parenteral antibiotics for severe cases with cellulitis
- Aspiration of lacrimal sac in a localized and pointing pyocele/mucocele - smear and cultures of the aspirate material and appropriate antibiotics

- Incision and drainage of a localized abscess and leaving the site open after packing the abscess cavity with antibiotics
- Dacryocystitis with total nasolacrimal duct (NLD) obstruction—wait till resolution of symptoms for at least a month and proceed with dacryocystorhinostomy (DCR).

CHRONIC DACRYOCYSTITIS

History

- History of recurrent episodes of watering with discharge
- History of any treatment taken
- History of previous lacrimal sac surgery
- History of acute episode of pain or swelling
- History of sinusitis, nasal obstruction
- History of dryness, grittiness and burning of the eyes
- History of drug intake
- History of radiation therapy.

Clinical Examination

- Swelling over the lacrimal sac region
- Presence of fistula with discharging mucoid or mucopurulent material
- Visual acuity
- Extraocular motility.

Examination in the Oculoplasty Department

- Position of the lids
- Look for matted lashes
- Tear film height
- Examination of the puncta
- ROPLAS test
- Diagnostic probing and irrigation of the upper lacrimal system

- *ENT evaluation:*
  - Nasal septal deviation
  - Hypertrophied and swollen turbinates
  - Nasal polyps
  - Nasal mass
  - Atrophic rhinitis
  - Sinusitis
- General health check up.

MANAGEMENT

External DCR/Endoscopic DCR.

Follow-up

- Relief of symptoms
- Wound integrity
- Periodic syringing in the postoperative period
- Suture removal generally on 5 to 7th postoperative day.

DACRYOCYSTOGRAPHY

It is the technique of imaging of the lacrimal drainage system by the injection of contrast material into the passages.

INDICATIONS
Complete Obstruction
- Determine exact location of obstruction
- Delineate anatomy in post-trauma patients and when reconstruction surgery is planned following failed lacrimal surgery
- When it is hard to differentiate between 'hard stop' and 'soft stop'
- Sac size determination for preoperative planning and prognosis estimation.

Incomplete Obstruction
- In patients with symptomatic epiphora, despite patency on irrigation of the lacrimal system
- Patients with suspected dacryoliths, lacrimal sac masses
- In combination with additional intervention like balloon dacryoplasty.

CONTRAINDICATIONS
- Contrast allergy
- Uncooperative patient.

PROCEDURE
- Detailed history including allergies to dye, etc. obtained
- Procedure is explained to the patient and informed consent obtained
- Patient asked to lie supine on a radiographic table
- Lacrimal sac palpated to detect any mass lesion or express any fluid present

- Topical anesthetic applied into conjunctival sac as drops or on cotton applicator over the lower punctum/canaliculus
- Lower punctum dilated
- Plain X-ray of the nasolacrimal drainage system taken
- Lower canaliculus cannulated with final metal/plastic cannula
- 0.5 to 1.0 cc contrast injection
- Radiographs usually taken at 0 minutes and 30 minutes.

Modifications
- Macrodacryocystography
- Digital subtraction dacryocystography
- Dacryocystofluoroscopy.

ENDOSCOPY

Endoscopy has diagnostic and therapeutic value in diseases of the lacrimal and orbital systems.

NASAL ENDOSCOPY

The patient's nostril should be packed with a nasal decongestant and topical anesthetic solution at least 15 minutes prior to the endoscopy.

It is mandatory prior to DCR surgery to assess for nasal pathology.

Presence of deviated nasal septum may be an indication for combined septoplasty if endoscopic DCR is planned.

Endoscopic DCR has the advantage of being more cosmetically appealing as it avoids an external scar and is recommended especially in young patients and in cases of lacrimal abscess.

Routine postoperative endoscopic examination with curettage and syringing is of importance in patients after endoscopic DCR. It is ideally done 1 week postoperatively and repeated after 6 weeks, and later as required.

Assessment of silastic tube within the nasal cavity can be done.

ENDOSCOPY IN ORBITAL SURGERY

It can be used for orbital decompression of the medial and inferior walls of the orbit (e.g. in cases of thyroid associated ophthalmopathy).

SOCKET EVALUATION

INSPECTION

- Presence of enophthalmos
- Superior sulcus deformity
- *Eyelids:*
  - Position
  - Lid laxity
  - Entropion, ectropion
  - Lagophthalmos
- Palpebral fissure
- Retention of prosthesis in the socket
- Sunken socket
- *Prosthesis:*
  - Scratches, roughened edges
  - Dried deposits
  - Motility
  - Cosmesis
- Socket after removal of prosthesis
- Health of the socket (conjunctival congestion or discharge)
- Fornices - contracture (mild, moderate or severe)
- Status of the orbital implant if present-whether well covered with conjunctiva or exposed, if exposed then amount of exposure to be noted.

PALPATION

- Intactness of orbital rims
- Any bony abnormality
- Any abnormal palpable mass within the socket
- Fitting of prosthesis.

  In children examination is done under anesthesia for evaluating the same.

MANAGEMENT

- Adequate fornices - try fitting a larger conformer or shell

- Marked enophthalmos—consider secondary implant
- Superior sulcus deformity—subperiosteal implantation is done
- Conjunctival shortage—mucous membrane graft and fornix forming sutures
- Severe contracture—dermis fat grafts, temporalis muscle transfer, etc.

Pre-and postoperative photographic documentation is necessary.

COUNSELING

- Take the patient into confidence
- Find out the expectations of the patient
- Emphasize the need for multiple surgeries for achieving the final outcome
- Give a realistic outcome of the surgery to the patient.

OCULAR PROSTHETIC DEPARTMENT

The hospital runs a special clinic, since 2000 for one eyed patients to help them rehabilitate with artificial eye. The department deals with creating hand made artificial eye called custom-made prosthesis (CMP) and readymade prosthesis. The department is managed by a trained Ocularist, who is a skilled technician trained in the art of painting, modifying and fitting an ocular prosthesis. In addition to creating it, the Ocularist shows the patient ways of handling, cleaning and taking care of their prosthesis, and provides long-term care through periodic examinations of the socket and prosthesis.

OCULAR PROSTHESIS

This is an artificial eye (shell) placed for cosmetic purposes.

The fitting of the prosthesis is done by the ocularist in conjunction with the oculoplasty department.

The prosthesis can be readymade (stock-eye) or custom-made.

Custom-made prosthesis gives the advantage of better cosmesis and motility as it tailor-made for the individual patient. Making of the prosthesis takes a minimum of three days and the patient is to be advised regarding the same. Measurements can also be taken in the operation theater, for example, when the patient is undergoing examination under GA. In these cases, the Ocularist is to informed the previous day.

Services Provided

Stock Shell

- Custom-made prosthesis
- Conformer
- Scleral shell.

Indications

- Enucleated eye
- Eviscerated eye
- Phthisical eye
- Anophthalmic/Microphthalmic eye.

Stock or Custom Prosthesis

The patients are generally seen by the Oculoplasty department doctors and referred for the Prosthesis department. As per the need of the eye condition, the fitting of stock or custom eye prosthesis is decided.

"Stock" or "readymade" ocular prostheses - Drawbacks: low grade acrylic, not made for any particular person, poor color match, and restricted movement.

"Custom" ocular prosthesis - high grade acrylic, biocompatible, better fit as it is hand-made, individualized for each person, good color match, better movement when compared with stock eye and allergies are unlikely.

Procedure

The impression of the socket is taken and a wax model is prepared.

Using the model, we determine the correct positioning of the iris, the outer curvature, and the extent to which the eyelids will open.

The wax model is then used to prepare a master mold which is filled with acrylic plastic to create a cast of the prosthesis.

The iris is hand painted from direct observation of the unaffected eye, including the sclera along with the blood vessels. It is then covered with a clear plastic protective coating and is cured once more. The prosthesis is now ready for a polishing to give it a perfectly smooth surface and wet-looking appearance.

Cleaning of Prosthesis

The stock shell is cleaned once a week and CMP once a month. Proper cleaning procedures should be followed. The proper way of cleaning the shell is washing with water and mild soap.

Complications

Watering of eyes, redness, discharge, pain, rotation of shell, itching can be avoided by following a proper cleaning schedule, decreasing frequency of handling of shell, and periodic polishing.

Follow-up

The ocular prosthesis needs to be polished regularly in order to restore the acrylic finish and ensure the health of the surrounding tissues. It is generally recommended that children between 3 to 9 years of age be seen every 6 months and all other patients at least once a year.

AESTHETIC CLINIC

It is a super specialty clinic run by the hospital. The clinic focuses on aesthetic and reconstructive aspects of the eyelids, the brows and the face. The commonly performed procedures are the repair of droopy eyelids and brows and rejuvenation procedures such as eyelid lifts, brow lifts, removal of eyelid bags, face and mid face lifts, liposuction and facial fat transfer. The clinic specializes in the minimally invasive procedures such as botox, dermal fillers, chemical peels, micro-dermabrasion of the skin, radiofrequency skin tightening and cosmeceuticals to correct the lines of aging, periocular skin pigmentation, dark circles for the overall facial rejuvenation.

DERMATOCHALASIS

Definition

The upper eyelids consist of extremely thin skin. As the eyelid skin stretches, it may show the first signs of aging on the face. Droopy upper eyelid skin with the eyelid bags due to the prolapsed orbtial fat pads is called dermatochalasis.

Management

It is corrected by a surgical rejuvunation procedure that removes an ellipse of excess skin and sculpting of the orbtial fat called blepharoplasty.

Indications

1. Dermatochalasis
2. Blepharochalasis

Examination

Basic examination has to be performed as it is done in a case of blepharoptosis.

Other parameters are:
1. Measurement of upper eyelid skin (minimum upper lid skin should be 20 mm).
2. Check for the elasticity of the skin.
3. Grading of the prolapsed fat pads (medial and central in upper eyelids, medial, central and lateral in the lower eyelids).
4. Eyelid laxity (distraction, snap test).

BROW PTOSIS

Definition

Aging changes in the brows can cause them to droop and lead to brow ptosis. It can be seen as tiredness, anger or sadness. The eyebrows can appear to sink or droop over time, due in part to stretching of skin and loss of fat that supports the brow. Brow droop can contribute to sagging of the upper eyelids called pseudodermatochalasis.

Management

The brow ptosis is corrected by the surgical procedure called brow ptosis repair. There are different types of repair and are tailored to the patients requirements and the amount of the brow ptosis present.

Indications

1. Brow ptosis.
2. Pseudodermatochalasis.

Examination

Basic examination has to be performed as it is done in a case of blepharoptosis and blepharoplasty.

Other parameters are:
Measurement of the brow ptosis (measured in mm by placing the ruler at 0 mark at the brow and the amount ptosis is measured by simulating the lift).

FACE AND MIDFACE LIFT

Definition

A facelift, technically known as a rhytidectomy is a type of cosmetic surgery procedure used to give a more youthful appearance. It usually involves the removal of excess facial skin, with or without the tightening of underlying tissues, and the redraping of the skin on the patient's face and neck.

In the traditional facelift, an incision is made in front of the ear extending up into the hairline. The incision curves around the bottom of the ear and then behind it, usually ending near the hairline on the back of the neck. After the skin incision is made, the skin is separated from the deeper tissues with a scalpel or scissors (also called undermining) over the cheeks and neck. At this point, the deeper tissues (SMAS, the fascial suspension system of the face) can be tightened with sutures, with or without removing some of the excess deeper tissues. The skin is then redraped, and the amount of excess skin to be removed is determined by the surgeon's judgment and experience. The excess skin is then removed, and the skin incisions are closed with sutures and staples.

Indications

1. Facial aging
2. Facial nerve paralysis.

Examination

1. Quality of the skin—texture, pigmentation and laxity.
2. Dynamic and the static wrinkles (forehead lines, glabellar lines, crows feet, marionette lines).
3. Facial folds (nasolabial folds).
4. Cheek droop and the loss of malar fat pads.
5. Jowls.
6. Platysmal bands.
7. Hairline.

AUTOLOGOUS FAT TRANSFER

Definition

Fat transfer (medically, fat transplantation, also called fat injection or fat grafting) is a medical procedure that uses the patient's own fat tissue to increase the volume of fat in the subcutaneous area of the body-face.

Fat is withdrawn from the patient in one of two ways: with a syringe that has a large-bore needle or with a liposuction cannula. The fat is prepared according to the practitioner's preferred method and then injected into the patient's recipient site. The preparation process clears the donor fat of blood and other unwanted ingredients that could cause infections or other undesirable side effects.

Indications

1. Facial aging and loss of facial fat.
2. Facial paralysis.
3. Enophthalmic sockets.

Examination

It is to be followed on same lines as in a patient for facelift.

BOTOX

Definition

Botox is a protein produced by the *Clostridium botulinum*. It is a nonsurgical treatment where it is injected directly into the muscles of facial expressions. It works by blocking nerve impulses to the injected muscles. This reduces muscle activity and smoothens the wrinkles/lines.

Indications

1. Forehead lines.
2. Glabellar lines.

3. Crows feet.
4. Perioral lines/smoke lines.
5. Marionette lines.
6. Dimpling of chin.
7. Platysmal bands.
8. Functional- Blepharospasm, hemifacial spasm, reflex lacrimation, gustatory tears.

DERMAL FILLERS

Definition

Dermal fillers are basically a collagen material made of synthetic or natural substances and is used for injection in the dermis for purposes of augmenting soft tissues, hence the facial rejuvenation.

Indications

1. Facial folds—nasolabial, tear trough deformity.
2. Static wrinkles.
2. Lips.
3. Cheek droop.
4. Scars and depressions.

2
Squint

- General Considerations
- History in Pediatric Patients
- Visual Acuity Estimation
- Refraction
- General Guidelines for Prescription of Glasses in Children
- Concomitant Squint
- General Guidelines for Management of Different Types of Concomitant Strabismus
- Incomitant Squint
- Congenital Cataract/Cataract in Children
- Nystagmus
- Contact Lens Fitting
- Contact Lens Clinic
- Contact Lens Related Problems
- Subluxated Lenses (Ectopia Lentis)
- Botulinum Toxin Injection

GENERAL CONSIDERATIONS

OUTPATIENT DEPARTMENT

- Children will be accompanied by an attendar at all times.
- Two attendars will be allowed with younger children and those with multiple handicaps and mentally retarded persons.
- Infants and younger children will get priority over adults in way of preliminary check up and consultation.

IN-PATIENT

- One attender per child will be allowed in general ward
- In private room two attenders will be allowed
- *Nil oral orders patients posted for general anesthesia will be as follows:*
    - *Solids:* Light meal/nonhuman milk – 6 hours
    - *Liquids:* Breast milk – 4 hours, infant formula, nonhuman milk - 6 hours
    - *Clear fluids:* (Water, fruit just without pulp, carbonated drinks) - 2 hours
- Any medication for systemic conditions should be kept with child.
- Keep the baby warm especially infants.
- For premature babies, include Theoped drops in premedication.
- All children, who require admission, to be admitted by 3 PM.
- Preoperative round and review by the anesthetist.
- High-risk consent will be taken by the ophthalmologist in outpatient department.

HISTORY IN PEDIATRIC PATIENTS

COMPLAINTS

- *Low vision:*
  - How and when was low vision noticed?
  - Does the child hold toys/books close to face? Complaints from the class teacher.
  - Does he respond to visual stimuli? Visual response in unfamiliar surroundings.
- *Squint:*
  - Unilateral or alternating or intermittent.
  - Any abnormal head posture, or abnormal movements.
  - When is the squint more noticeable?
  - Is it related to fatigue or illness?
  - Any diplopia?
  - Precipitating factors like trauma, febrile episode before onset of squint.

PAST HISTORY

- Previous treatment, spectacles, occlusion, drops, surgery.
- Associated complaints like photophobia, epiphora, pain, redness.

BIRTH AND MEDICAL HISTORY

- Gestational age
- Significant antenatal history
- Maternal infection, any drugs taken during pregnancy
- History of any other handicap
- Any untoward event during delivery
- Birth trauma, forceps, birth asphyxia
- Birth weight of the child
- History of being kept in incubator
- History of oxygenation

- Is the child thriving well?
- Developmental milestones, both physical and mental
- Any associated systemic problem
- Other associated neurological problems like cerebral palsy, epilepsy, mental retardation and craniofacial anomalies.

FAMILY HISTORY

- Consanguinity
- Similar problems in other siblings
- History of any inherited eye or systemic condition.

VISUAL ACUITY ESTIMATION

INFANTS AND TODDLERS

- Fixation pattern
- Resistance to occlusion of either eye
- Visually evoked potential (VEP)
- Optokinetic nystagmus testing
- Preferential looking tests like Teller cards
- Doll's eye maneuver.

PRELITERATE CHILDREN

- Allen cards
- Lea symbols
- Landolt C and Tumbling E
- Sheridan Gardiner test
- If unable to record vision a copy of the chart can be given to the parent to train the child at home.

SCHOOL-GOING CHILDREN

- Lea symbols
- Snellen
- Landolt C and Tumbling E.

PATIENTS WITH NYSTAGMUS

- Record monocular as well as binocular vision
- Fog the contralateral eye without occluding it when recording monocular vision. High plus lens can be use to fog the contralateral eye
- Record vision with preferred head posture, if any.

REFRACTION

- Do subjective refraction if possible
- Do cycloplegic refraction in all patients reporting to the pediatric ophthalmology clinic.

CHOICE OF CYCLOPLEGIC AGENT

- *Atropine 1 percent ointment 3 times a day × 3 days:*
  - Recommended in accommodative esotropia, accommodative spasm, varying retinoscopy values
  - Maximum cycloplegic effect – 3 to 6 hours
  - Lasts for two weeks.
- *Cyclopentolate 1 percent drops. In children above 3 years, instill 2 times at an interval of 5 minutes:*
  - Maximum cycloplegic effect 20 to 45 minutes
  - Do refraction after 30 minutes
  - Lasts for 1 to 3 days.
- *Homatropine 2 to 5 percent recommended in children over 3 years of age:*
  - Maximum cycloplegic effect 25 to 45 minutes
  - Do refraction after 30 minutes
  - Last 2 to 3 days.
- For cyclopentolate-tropicamide-cyclopentolate (CTC) flash, 1 drop of 1 percent cyclopentolate is instilled at 5 minutes interval, followed by 1 drop of 0.5 percent tropicamide, again followed by instillation of 1 percent cyclopentolate at 5 minutes interval.
- Perform a cycloplegic refraction between 45 and 75 minutes after the last drop instillation (the minimum wait time of 45 minutes ensures all iris colors are in maximal cycloplegia before refraction).
- If the cycloplegic refraction cannot be performed between 45 and 75 minutes, instill another drop of cyclopentolate 1.0 percent in each eye and wait a minimum of 30 minutes more.

- For homatropine (HA) and tropicamide (T) flash, 1 drop of homatropine 2 percent is applied followed by 1 drop of 0.5 percent tropicamide at 5 minutes interval.

The CTC flash or HA and T flash can be carried out appropriately in all new patients below 12 years of age, and in all children with refractive errors detected for the first time.

Note

- *Adverse reactions to cycloplegic agents:*
  - *Atropine:* Dryness of mouth, flushing, irritability, fever
  - *Cyclopentolate:* Gastrointestinal disturbance and transient psychosis
  - *Homatropine:* Same as atropine.
- *Children with light colored eyes and infants may need modification of dose.*
- *In premature babies and infants below 6 months of age dose should be modified.*
- *Avoid atropine in Down's syndrome, cerebral palsy, trisomy 13, 18 and other central nervous system (CNS) disorders.*
- *Cyclopentolate is contraindicated in children with seizures, mental retardation, cerebral palsy and other neurological abnormalities.*

METHOD

- Do retinoscopy after maximum cycloplegia is achieved.
- Darken the room to avoid distraction.
- Child can fixate on retinoscope light.
- Use loose lenses to neutralize the reflex.
- Postmydriatic test—to be done in older children.

GENERAL GUIDELINES FOR PRESCRIPTION OF GLASSES IN CHILDREN

MYOPIA

- Give full correction including cylinder
- Contact lenses, in high myopes, to avoid image minification may be prescribed in older children
- Avoid overcorrection of myopia in orthophoric children
- Do not prescribe myopic correction without a cycloplegic refraction.

HYPEROPIA

- Insignificant hyperopia, i.e. up to +3.0, in the absence of esotropia or reduced vision, can be left uncorrected
- If there is an esodeviation full cycloplegic correction is prescribed
- In school-going children, less than full cycloplegic correction could be prescribed, to avoid distance blur, even if there is esotropia
- Hyperopia may be corrected, even if insignificant, if there is a strong family history of accommodative esotropia.

ASTIGMATISM

- Visually significant astigmatism should be fully corrected
- Insignificant astigmatism in very young children can be left undercorrected
- Refine the cylinder using Jackson's cross cylinder wherever possible.

CONSENSUS GUIDELINES FOR PRESCRIBING EYEGLASSES IN YOUNG CHILDREN

Myopia

- *Isometropia:*
  - Prescribe if ≥– 4.00 D in children less than 2 years
  - Children 2 to 3 years, prescribe if ≥ –3.00 D.
- In cases of anisometropia, prescribe if the difference is ≥ –2.50 D.

Hyperopia

- *Esotropia:*
  - In children < 1 year prescribe if ≥ + 3.00 D.
  - Older children ≥ + 2.00 D.
- *No deviation:*
  - In infants, give glasses if hyperopia ≥ + 5.00 D.
  - In children 2 to 3 years, prescribe for ≥ 4.50 D.
- In cases of anisometropia, prescribe if ≥ 2.00 D.

Astigmatism

- In younger children, prescribe if ≥ 3.00 and in > 2 to 3 years age if ≥ 2.00 D
- In cases of anisometropia prescribe if ≥ 2.00 D.

AMBLYOPIA

Amblyopia is a unilateral or, less commonly, bilateral reduction of best corrected visual acuity that cannot only and directly be attributed to the effect of a structural abnormality of the eye or the visual pathways. It is a diagnosis of exclusion. Amblyopia is caused by abnormal visual experience early in life resulting from one of the following:

- Strabismus
- Anisometropia or high bilateral refractive errors (isometropia)
- Visual deprivation.

DIAGNOSTIC CRITERIA FOR AMBLYOPIA

Criterion	Finding
Unilateral amblyopia	
Fixation preference	Unequal fixation behavior
Preferential looking	2 octave difference
Best corrected visual acuity	≥ 2 line (Snellen) difference
Bilateral amblyopia	Vision < 20/40 each eye

In the Amblyopia Treatment Study Group trials, **mild-to-moderate amblyopia** is defined as visual acuity in the amblyopic eye of 20/80 or better. **Severe amblyopia** is defined as visual acuity in the amblyopic eye of 20/100 to 20/400.

Management

- Success rates decline with increasing age
- All children should be considered for treatment of amblyopia. In older children (up to 17 years of age) occlusion can be tried provided it has not been tried before.

Prognosis depends on:
- Age of the patient at detection
- Cause and severity of amblyopia
- History of previous treatment
- Duration of amblyopia
- Compliance with treatment.

CHOICE OF THERAPY

The following therapies are used alone or in combination as required to achieve the therapeutic goal.
- Optical correction
- *Occlusion:* With adhesive patches—full time or part time patching depending on the age and severity of amblyopia
- *Penalization:* With atropine 1 percent eyedrops.

CONCOMITANT SQUINT

HISTORY

- Age of onset of squint
- Precipitating factors like trauma, febrile illness
- Associated abnormal eye movements or abnormal head position
- Symptoms of asthenopia
- Double vision
- Eye closure in bright light
- Previous surgery for strabismus
- Occlusion therapy and compliance
- Previous spectacle wear
- Application of drops like phospholine iodide
- Any other surgery like retinal detachment (RD), cataract, glaucoma implant, sinus surgery or neuro-surgery.

BIRTH HISTORY AND MEDICAL HISTORY (SEE SECTION 2.1)

Family History

- Consanguinity
- Strabismus
- Response of other members of family to surgery
- High ametropia.

External Examination

- Shape of head
- Facial asymmetry
- Dysmorphic facial features like sparse hair, frontal bossing
- Ear abnormalities
- Any other deformities like extra digits
- General appearance including obesity.

Examination

- Record visual acuity for near and distance
- Do retinoscopy and subjective refraction
- Note any abnormal head posture like head tilt, face turn etc
- Assess lid position—note any ptosis, lid retraction.
- Do a cover test, cover uncover and alternate cover test
- Hirschberg's test in case of uncooperative patients and those with poor fixation/vision
- Note any nystagmus – mention type of nystagmus, jerk or pendular, note null point if any
- Check ductions and versions
- Note any limitation, overaction and underaction of muscles.

ANTERIOR SEGMENT EXAMINATION BY SLIT-LAMP/TORCH LIGHT

- Note any congenital anomalies like aniridia, coloboma, heterochromia, cataract
- Check pupillary reaction.

In the Squint Clinic

- Review history.
- Sensory evaluation has to be done before motor evaluation.
- *Check binocular sensory status:*
    - *Stereopsis:* Use Titmus fly/Lang's chart
    - *Retinal correspondence:* Use Bagolini's glasses/ Worth four dot test/Synaptophore
    - *Suppression:* Worth four dot test/Bagolini's glasses.
- Confirm presence or absence of abnormal head posture.
- Confirm the findings of cover tests.
- Measure angle of deviation near and distance, with and without glasses.

- Use Krimsky's test/Hirschberg's test in uncooperative patients and those with poor fixation.
- Check ductions and versions.
- Note A or V or X pattern if any.
- Perform additional tests if indicated, like measurement of AC/A ratio, 4Δ Base out test, fusional amplitudes, forced duction test.
- Do cycloplegic refraction.
- Fundus examination (Note any torsion suggestive of oblique overaction).

MANAGEMENT

- Correct refractive error by appropriate glasses
- Manage amblyopia by occlusion regimen.

Penalization

- Atropine eyedrops 1 percent once in a week. Instruct parents about possible side effects of atropine.
- Tropicamide 1 percent eyedrops once a day.

Occlusion

- By a patch or frosted glasses depending on the visual acuity level, presence of binocularity and compliance.
- Part time in cases of mild anisometropic amblyopia, or where follow-up is likely to be poor, or compliance with full time occlusion is less likely. Part-time occlusion is also useful for maintenance after discontinuing full time occlusion.
- Follow-up patients every month if on full time occlusion.

Surgery

Plan surgery, if indicated, only when vision has equalized or there is spontaneous good alternation, or if there is no improvement in vision even after a full aggressive trial of amblyopia therapy.

GENERAL GUIDELINES FOR MANAGEMENT OF DIFFERENT TYPES OF CONCOMITANT STRABISMUS

INFANTILE ESOTROPIA

- Plan surgery early, eyes should be aligned by age 24 months to optimize binocular cooperation.
- Ensure free alternation before surgery.
- Goal of treatment is alignment within 8 prism diopter of orthotropia with at least peripheral fusion.
- Do bilateral medial rectus recession according to angle of deviation with inferior oblique weakening procedures if there is associated inferior oblique overaction.
- Follow-up at six weeks and every six months.

ACCOMMODATIVE ESOTROPIA

- Give full cycloplegic correction
- Delay in initiation of treatment increases the likelihood of not responding to antiaccommodative therapy
- Treat amblyopia
- Gradually decrease hyperopic correction if good control of ensuing esophoria
- Can try phospholine iodide in cases of poor compliance with glasses. Instruct parents about possible side effects
- Follow-up frequently if on phospholine iodide.

PARTIALLY ACCOMMODATIVE ESOTROPIA

- Give full cycloplegic correction.
- Treat amblyopia.
- Be conservative about planning surgery.
- Rule out latent uncorrected hyperopia before proceeding with surgery

- Do a bilateral medial rectus recession for residual angle of deviation over full cycloplegic correction.
- Plan undercorrection.
- Explain to parents that the child needs to wear glasses even after surgery.

ESOTROPIA WITH HIGH AC/A RATIO

- Give full cycloplegic correction.
- Treat amblyopia if any.
- Prescribe executive bifocals bisecting the pupil if distance deviation is less that 15Δ.
- Acceptable response is fusion at distance with less than 10 prism diopter of residual esotropia through bifocal at near fixation .
- Can use phopholine iodide.
- Plan bilateral medial rectus recession if distance deviation is more than 15Δ even with glasses.

INTERMITTENT DIVERGENT SQUINT

- Prescribe corrective lenses for refractive errors
- Myopia and astigmatism should be fully corrected
- Ignore hyperopia of up to +2.00 D
- High hyperopia > 4 D needs to be corrected as optical blur may itself
- Increase exotropia
- Assess stereopsis
- Measure squint angle for both near and distance
- Rule out pseudo divergence excess if angle is more for distance than near by controlling fusion and accommodation
- Observe if measurement of deviation is unreliable or if child is able to control deviation well
- Over minus lens effective as temporary measure to delay surgery in preschool age children
- Surgical correction depending on the angle of the deviation.

- *Indication for surgery:*
  - Increase in the angle of deviation with deteriorating control
  - Decrease in stereoacuity
  - Coexisting convergence insufficiency refractory to orthoptic treatment
  - Asthenopia
  - Development of amblyopia/suppression.

INCOMITANT SQUINT

HISTORY

- Diplopia—duration, mode of onset, diurnal variation
- Abnormal head posture
- Trauma
- Systemic conditions like DM, IHD, thyroid disorder
- Abnormal eye movements
- Oscillopsia, if nystagmus is present
- Associated neurological symptoms like loss of consciousness, convulsion, motor weakness, slurring of speech, giddiness, etc.

EXAMINATION

- Record visual acuity *(refer to 2.1 to 2.4)*
- Do dynamic retinoscopy
- Note any abnormal head posture
- Do cover tests
- Note difference between primary and secondary deviation
- Check versions and ductions
- Note limitation, overaction and underaction of muscles.

AT SQUINT CLINIC

- Review history
- Note any anomalous head posture, position of lids
- Perform cover tests
- Measure angle of deviation both primary and secondary, in all cardinal positions of gaze
- In adults assess if single binocular vision is achieved in primary position and reading position with prisms
- Recheck ductions and versions
- Check torsion by Maddox rod/Double Maddox rod
- Do diplopia charting/Hess charting

- Do Park's three step test in case of vertical strabismus
- Perform forced duction test if indicated
- Detailed fundus evaluation
- Neuroimaging in cases of recent onset paralytic strabismus in the absence of diabetes, hypertension, in cases of trauma, or when multiple cranial neuropathies or suspected space-occupying lesion
- Order thyroid function tests and rule out myasthenia, when etiology is unclear
- Order cross consultation with neuro-ophthalmologist if indicated.

MANAGEMENT

- Observation if paralysis is of acute onset
- Botulinum toxin injection into the antagonist muscle in selected cases
- Patch to relieve diplopia
- Prisms to achieve binocular vision in case of small angle deviation
- Do surgery in patients with large angle deviation, after waiting for at least six months after the onset, for recovery and stability. Surgical plan is based on Hess charting, measured angle of deviation. Adjustable suture technique is better as results are unpredictable.

CONGENITAL CATARACT/ CATARACT IN CHILDREN

HISTORY

- When was white reflex noted?
- Congenital cataract in the family—sibling history
- Trauma/child abuse
- Redness, pain before cataract
- Behavioral pattern of child at home, school
- Visual status—ambulation in familiar and unfamiliar surroundings
- School performance, especially reading.

Birth History

- History of and degree of consanguinity
- Maternal infection especially 1st trimester of pregnancy
- Gestational age
- Birth weight
- Birth trauma, untoward event during delivery
- Supplemental O_2 therapy or being kept in incubator
- Developmental milestones
- Feeding/digestive behavior
- Developmental anomalies.

EXAMINATION

Visual Function

- Assess fixation, fixation behavior, fixation preference, objection to occlusion
- Record visual acuity and fixation pattern in older children
- Refraction
- Do cover test/Hirschberg's test to detect strabismus
- Note nystagmus if any

Strabismus and nystagmus are late signs that cataract is visually significant.

Slit-Lamp Examination

- Look for any congestion
- Evidence of recent or old trauma like corneal opacity, iris hole, anterior chamber (AC) reaction ruptured anterior capsule, lens matter in AC, etc.
- Associated congenital anomalies like iris coloboma, lens coloboma, corneal opacities, microcornea
- Note irregularly deep anterior chamber. Do Gonioscopy if child cooperates in cases of traumatic cataract
- Look for evidence of inflammation like keratic precipitates, AC reaction, peripheral anterior synechiae
- Pupillary reaction, look for any relative afferent pupillary defect (RAPD)
- Mention type of cataract, zonular, PSC, traumatic, posterior lenticonus, persistent hyperplastic primary vitreous (PHPV)
- Rule out any foreign body
- Note any iridodonesis, or phacodonesis or sub-luxation of lens
- Check intraocular pressure by Tonopen, Applanation if indicated
- Do fundus examination if the cataract allows
- It is very important to rule out other causes of leukocoria like retinoblastoma, endophthalmitis, Coats' disease.

INVESTIGATIONS

- Ultrasound (USG) if fundus view is not possible, to assess posterior segment, and to rule out posterior mass, retinal detachment, optic nerve stalk to lens, intraocular foreign body in traumatic cataract
- CT scan if intraocular foreign body is suspected and not seen on USG
- Rule out TORCH and inborn errors of metabolism by lab tests in congenital cataract
- Ultrasound biomicroscopy if zonular integrity is suspect

- Any further work up should be directed by other abnormalities in growth and development, with input from geneticist, metabolic expert, or dysmorphologist.

MANAGEMENT
Indications for Surgery

- Poor vision
- Drop in school performance
- Development of a squint, which was previously not there
- Development of nystagmus.

Surgical Management

All children should undergo a detailed ocular examination of corneal diameter, intraocular pressure, axial length, angle assessment with direct goniolens, pachymetry, keratometry under anesthesia prior to surgery.

Unilateral Cataract

- Below 6
  months of age : Lensectomy
- Above 6
  months of age : Phacoemulsification +
                   Intraocular lens implantation +
                   Primary posterior
                   capsulotomy + anterior
                   vitrectomy

IOL to be deferred if axial length is less than 18 mm or corneal diameter is less than 10 mm or if there is a pre-existing ocular comorbidity .

Bilateral Cataract

- Below 12   : Lensectomy
  months of age
- More than 12 : Phacoemulsification +
  months of age   Intraocular lens implantation +
                   Primary posterior
                   capsulotomy + Anterior vitrectomy

Older cooperative children could have a Yag laser capsulotomy instead of a primary posterior capsulotomy + anterior vitrectomy.

Early Intraocular Lens Implantation

Various studies currently have concluded that carefully and meticulously performed primary IOL implantation appears to be a safe and effective method of aphakic correction in children younger than one year of age. PPC and anterior vitrectomy reduces the rate of secondary opacification of the visual axis in a pseudophakic eye. Hence, primary IOL implantation can be considered for infants with normal corneal diameter and average axial length.

POSTOPERATIVE FOLLOW-UP

- Close follow-up in the immediate postoperative period.
- Manage inflammation with aggressive topical steroid and cycloplegic.
- Use topical antibiotics in case of traumatic cataract.

VISUAL REHABILITATION

- Fit contact lenses for unilateral aphakia.
- Give glasses for bilateral aphakia. Glass prescription may be for near correction.
- Bifocal to be prescribed once child is about to start school.
- Treat amblyopia if indicated.
- Squint correction later if needed.
- Genetic counseling if a strong family history of congenital cataract.
- Periodic follow-up visits for change of glasses, monitoring for complications like secondary glaucoma, posterior capsular opacification, optic capture, retinal detachment.

NYSTAGMUS

HISTORY

- Congenital or acquired
- History of oscillopsia
- Visual behavior of child
- History of poor vision
- Any associated abnormal head posture
- Any neurological problem
- History of photophobia
- Family history of similar problems.

EXAMINATION

- Visual acuity *(refer to 2.1 – 2.4)*
- Binocular visual acuity in the preferred head posture
- Monocular vision by avoiding occlusion, i.e. fogging
- Visual acuity for near
- Note head posture
- *Nystagmus:* Jerk/pendular, frequency, amplitude, uniplanar/multiplanar
- Anterior segment examination—especially iris structure, look for transillumination defects to rule out albinism, aniridia, iris coloboma
- Pupil—look for (RAPD), anisocoria, paradoxical pupillary response
- Ocular motility—look for strabismus which is due to poor vision or attempt too converge to dampen nystagmus
- Color vision
- *Fundus examination:* Optic disc examination, foveal reflex, pigment abnormalities.

INVESTIGATIONS

- *Electroretinogram (ERG):* In many patients with normal appearing posterior poles, ERG may be necessary to identify the cause.
- *Neuroimaging.*

Indications

- Poor vision with normal ERG and abnormal optic nerve
- Vertical nystagmus
- Atypical nystagmus like seesaw nystagmus
- Acquired nystagmus.

MANAGEMENT

Optical

- Correct refractive error
- Treat amblyopia—risk factors for amblyopia are anisometropia, astigmatism
- Prefer penalization instead of occlusion for amblyopia therapy
- Over minus lenses to reduce amplitude of nystagmus
- Prisms
- Contact lenses
- Low vision aid (LVA).

Surgical Correction

Goals of surgery are:
- To abolish anomalous head posture.
- To improve visual acuity.

Kestenbaum-Anderson procedure is the procedure of choice.

CONTACT LENS FITTING

- Find out if patient is aware about contact lenses
- Check if patient is an older user
- If a user, find out the type of lens used
- Ask if any problems with the lens
- Explain about contact lenses to patient and attendant
- Explain need for contact lenses
- Explain time required for dispensing
- Check if patient is interested
- Explain about the cost and maintenance of contact lenses
- Decide on type of lens to fit.

INDICATIONS
Soft Lens

- Astigmatism <1.50 D
- The astigmatism ≤ 1/3 of the sphere power
- Patient is unable to tolerate rigid gas permeable (RGP) lenses
- Patient is keen on soft lenses only
- Patient is a previous soft lens user.

Rigid Gas Permeable Lens

- Astigmatism >1.50 D
- Irregular corneal surfaces
- Corneal opacities
- Keratoconus.

Hard Lens

- Specified as hard trial
- Very high astigmatism.

CONTRAINDICATIONS

- Active infection or inflammation
- Inability to handle the contact lens.

CONTACT LENS TRIAL STEPS

- K reading
- Decide on base curve
- Fit the contact lens
- Adaptation time of 15 to 30 minutes (or till tearing subsides)
- Check fit
- Over refraction
- Decide on final contact lens parameters
- Send patient for payment
- Fill in order form
- Give the file for ordering of the lens
- Contact lens (CL) teaching to be given
- Hand over lens + kit to the patient.

RIGID GAS PERMEABLE LENS (SEMI SOFT LENS) FITTING

- Take the K reading: K1 @ axis, K2 @ axis
- The base curve (BC) is the flatter K
- Power of trial lens to be within 4 D of required power
- Fit the lens
- Adaptation time—till tearing subsides
- *Check the fit pattern:*
  - Centration of the lens
  - Movement in different gazes
  - Movement with blink
  - Fluorescein pattern assessment
- If the fit is good, then do an over refraction
- Decide final lens parameter
- Dispense lens.

Steep Fit

Symptoms

- Vision will be better after a blink
- Initially will be comfortable, will get painful towards the end of the day
- Difficult to remove
- Pain on removal.

Signs

- Indentation ring
- Peripheral corneal vascularization.

Management

Alter Fit by:
- Flattening base curve (e.g. if 7.5 mm steep, then 7.7 mm)
- Decrease the diameter.

Flat Fit

Symptoms

- Vision better before blink
- Does not stay on the eye
- Excessive movement.

Signs

- Central corneal staining
- Scratch marks on the cornea centrally.

Management

Alter Fit by:
- Steepening BC (e.g. if 7.7 mm flat, then 7.5 mm)
- Increasing diameter.

CONTACT LENS CLINIC

SOFT CONTACT LENS FITTING

Steps

- Obtain K reading : K1 @ axis, K2 @ axis
- Base curve = Flatter K in mm +1.0 mm
- *Choose appropriate power:* If power >± 4.00 Ds consider vertex conversion
- Fit the lenses
- Adaptation time to be given
- *Check fit:*
  - Centration
  - Movement
  - Limbal coverage
  - Push up test
- If fit good then over refraction
- Decide final lens
- Fill in order form
- Teaching to be given
- Lens and kit to be handed over.

FOLLOW-UP EXAMINATION/AFTER CARE

History

1. Vision with lenses
2. Comfort with lenses
3. Handling
   - Hands washed with soap?
     - What type of soap
     - Drying of the hands
   - Insertion and Removal—what is done to the lens after removal?
   - How is the lens stored?
     - Solution used
     - Any other solution used
   - Lens case cleaning
   - *Wearing schedule followed:*

  - Time of insertion
  - Time of removal
  - Any break in between
  - Number of days the lenses are worn continuously
- Age of lens case
- What is done to the lens case after wearing the lens
- Is tap water used for any particular purpose?

Examination

1. Vision with contact lenses.
2. Fit of the lens.
   - Centration
   - Movement
   - Fluorescein pattern/limbal coverage.
3. Slit-lamp examination of the cornea/conjunctiva.
4. Fluorescein examination of cornea SPKs, staining.
5. Lens examination
   - Edge
   - Color
   - Deposits
   - Shape of the lens.

CONTACT LENS RELATED PROBLEMS

CONTACT LENS-INDUCED PAPILLARY CONJUNCTIVITIS

Etiology

Immune response.

Symptoms

- Mucus formation, itching
- Wor se on contact lens removal
- Lens intolerance
- Greasy lenses.

Management

- Discontinue contact lens
- Improve hygiene
- Change cleaning system if needed
- Increase the frequency of lens change.

BULBAR CONJUNCTIVAL HYPEREMIA

Etiology

- Solution allergy
- Edema
- Hypoxia
- Dry eye
- Environmental
- Infection
- Poor fit
- Deposits.

Symptoms

- Increased contact lens intolerance
- Burning
- Itching.

Management

Remove source of problem.

LIMBAL HYPEREMIA

Etiology

- Hypoxia, tight lens
- Atopy, allergic reactions
- Toxic solution reactions
- Poor lens fit.

Symptoms

Depends on cause, pain may be none to severe.

Management

- If symptoms present. Cease lens wear until resolution
- Alleviation of cause.

CORNEAL STAINING

Etiology

- Mechanical, foreign body in CL exposure, disruption of tear film
- Metabolic, hypoxia, toxic/allergic reaction.

Symptoms

Normally asymptomatic.

Management

- Remove lenses for 1 to 3 days
- Stop at least 7 days of CL wear if immediate and widespread stromal diffusion of fluorescein exists
- If recurrent, change causative agent
- Advise to use saline instead of water to clean lens
- Medical treatment for corneal staining involving more than 1/3rd of the cornea
- Change fit or CL if required.

SUPERIOR ARCUATE STAINING
Etiology
Mechanical pressure of lens on cornea.

Symptoms
Symptomatic with CL removal and insertion.

Management
As for corneal staining: Remove lens for 7 days and replace lens with better fit or design or material.

3 AND 9 O'CLOCK STAINING
Etiology
Found in RGP lenses due to bad lens design, thick lens edge, tight lens, insufficient blink, too small lens.

Symptoms
Lens intolerance.

Management
- Change lens design to optimize edge design
- Blinking exercises.

CORNEAL EDEMA
Etiology
Lack of oxygen across the whole cornea.

Symptoms
None or blue vision.

Management
Increase oxygen and stop extended wear.

CENTRAL CORNEAL CLOUDING
Etiology
Fluid accumulation in edematous cornea.

Symptoms

Visual disturbance after lens removal and haloes.

Management

Increase oxygen, maintain lens wear.

DEPOSITS

Etiology

Hydrophobic spot on lens leading to a build-up of lens calcium, protein and lipid.

Symptoms

Discomfort and blurred vision.

Management

- New lens required
- Review surfactant cleaning procedure
- Increase replacement frequency
- Change lens material. Move to RGP or disposable
- Cleaning regimen—protein removal.

SUBLUXATED LENSES (ECTOPIA LENTIS)

DEFINITION

Partial displacement of lens from its normal position, secondary to congenital or acquired zonular weakness.

COMMON CONDITIONS ASSOCIATED WITH ECTOPIA LENTIS

Ocular

- Aniridia
- Iris coloboma
- Trauma
- Hereditary ectopia lentis
- Congenital glaucoma.

Systemic Conditions

- Marfan's syndrome
- Homocystinuria
- Weil Marchesani syndrome
- Hyperlysinemia
- Ehlers-Danlos syndrome.

HISTORY

- Low vision
- Squint
- Nystagmus
- Trauma.

Medical History

- Associated systemic feature
- Milestones.

Family History

Of other family members with similar condition.

CLINICAL EXAMINATION

- Refract the phakic and aphakic part
- Ocular motility examination for strabismus
- *Slit-lamp examination:*
  - Note direction of subluxation
  - Zonular status-elongated, torn or absent
  - Status of clarity of lens
  - How much pupillary area is phakic
  - Other associated ocular anomalies
  - In cases of trauma look for other sequelae of trauma
- Fundus examination.

Work-up

- Systemic examination by a pediatrician to rule out other systemic association
- Screening for inborn errors of metabolism
- Urine HPLC test for homocystinuria
- Echocardiogram
- Ultrasound biomicroscopy to evaluate zonular status.

MANAGEMENT

- Genetic counseling
- Special investigation
- Give best possible refractive correction by glasses/ contact lens
- Correct amblyopia
- *Indications for surgery:*
  - Cataractous lens
  - Anteriorly subluxated lens which may compromise cornea or cause increase in intraocular pressure
  - Posteriorly dislocated lens
  - Large myopic astigmatism
  - Asymmetric optical correction
- *Surgical options:*
  - Lensectomy with or without scleral fixated intraocular lens in cases where zonular loss is

high. Scleral fixation of intraocular lens not recommended in children below seven years of age

- Phacoemulsification with intraocular lens implantation with endocapsular ring in case of localized zonular damage.

BOTULINUM TOXIN INJECTION

It is frozen lyophilized form of toxin produced by *Clostridium botulinum*. Out of six toxins produced by *Clostridium botulinum*, type A is used clinically.

MECHANISM OF ACTION

Produces temporary, reversible, dose-related paralysis of, when injected into the muscle. It acts by inhibiting release of acetylcholine at presynaptic nerve terminals of cholinergic axons.

Available commercial preparations:
- Oculinum
- Dysport
- Botox.

CLINICAL USES

- Strabismus
- Blepharospasm
- Hemifacial spasm
- Nystagmus
- Miscellaneous.

RECONSTITUTION

2.5 units per 0.1 ml.

INJECTION PROCEDURE

- Take informed consent
- Explain procedure
- Injection made subcutaneously at sites depending on muscles that need to be paralyzed
- Rule out secondary causes of blepharospasm such as dry eyes and foreign body
- Essential blepharospasm needs no neuroimaging prior to injection

- Hemifacial spasm needs neuroimaging prior to injection
- Extraocular muscles are injected with EMG control.

POSSIBLE SIDE EFFECTS

- Ptosis
- Watering
- Subconjunctival hemorrhage
- Retrobulbar hemorrhage
- Induced deviation.

3

Cornea

- Outpatient Department Procedures
- Infective Conjunctivitis
- Corneal Foreign Body
- Ocular Allergy – Allergic Conjunctivitis
- Vernal Catarrh/Allergic Conjunctivitis
- Exposure Keratopathy
- Giant Papillary Conjunctivitis
- Band-shaped Keratopathy
- Pterygium
- Corneal Infections
- Corneal Opacity
- Dermoid
- Corneal Ectasia
- Corneal Dystrophy
- Corneal Graft Rejection
- Ocular Surface Disease
- Ocular Surface Squamous Neoplasia

OUTPATIENT DEPARTMENT PROCEDURES

CONJUNCTIVAL SWAB

Purpose

Conjunctival swab is done to look for microorganisms causing conjunctivitis. It is indicated in *ophthalmia neonatorum*, hyperacute conjunctivitis, conjunctivitis in immediate postoperative period, blebed eyes, suspected chlamydial conjunctivitis and chronic conjunctivitis of unknown etiology(follicular conjunctivitis or membranous conjunctivitis require conjunctival scrapping).

Procedure

After explaining to the patient under topical anesthesia the sterile cotton tipped application is used to sweep the conjunctival surface (usually the inferior fornix) and handed over to the technician from the Microbiology laboratory.

CORNEAL SCRAPPING

Purpose

This is done under topical anesthesia as an OPD procedure by the cornea specialist to look for the organism causing corneal infection. It is indicated in active infectious keratitis and chronic nonhealing keratitis and also a sudden nonresponse to previously responding keratitis to treatment.

Procedure

After explaining to the patient under topical anesthesia a 15 No. blade is used to gently scrape off material from the base of the ulcer and subjected to microbiological examination.

ROUTINE SMEARS

- Grams : Bacteria
- KOH : Fungus
- Giemsa : Cytology
- Immunofluroscent stain : Virus, *Chlamydia*

The smear report should be reviewed on the same day.

ROUTINE CULTURES

- Blood agar : All organisms (fastidious and non-fastidious)
- Chocolate agar : *Haemophilus*
- MacConkeys agar : Enteric organisms
- Brucella blood agar : Anaerobic organisms
- Sabouraud's dextrose agar : Fungus
- Brain-heart infusion broth : Aerobic organisms
- Thioglycolate broth : Anaerobic organisms

The culture report should also to be followed up at regular intervals starting from 24 to 48 hours.

Special Culture

- Lowenstein Jenson medium—*Mycobacterium tuberculosis*
- Nonnutrient agar with *E. coli overlay*—*Acanthamoeba*.

Corneal scrapping is not to be done in healing ulcers, only very deep infiltrates without epithelial defects. In severe corneal thinning which is impending perforation, corneal scrapping can be done gently.

SCHIRMER'S TEST

This is to access the aqueous component of tear.

Test 1

Procedure

Whatman No. 14 filter paper is used. The paper is bent at the notch and is inserted in the fornix at the junction of the medial 2/3 and lateral 1/3 of the lower eyelid in both the eyes. Care must be taken not to touch the cornea. The patient may keep the eyes open or closed. The length of the strip, which is become wet at the end of 5 minutes is measured.

Result
More than 10 mm wetting at the end of 5 minutes is as taken as normal.

Test 2

Procedure
The test may be repeated after a drop of local anesthetic is instilled into the cul-de-sac and drying it with a cotton bud. The amount of wetting at the end of 5 minutes gives a measurement of basal tear secretion.

Result
5 mm wetting in 5 minutes is taken as normal.

Reflex Secretion

Procedure
The ipsilateral nasal mucosa is stimulated with a cotton bud and the Schirmers test is repeated as above.

Result
Normal reflective secretion is more than 5 mm of wetting in 5 minutes.

PUNCTAL OCCLUSION

Definition

Punctal occlusion is a procedure that involves occlusion of the lacrimal puncta leading to the canaliculi, nasolacrimal sac and duct, to preserve existing scanty tear production in the management of dry eyes. Punctal occlusion can be performed either with temporary occlusive devices or with permanent occlusive devices or procedures.

Types

Temporary Occlusion

- The procedure is usually performed under magnification, with patient seated on the slit lamp.
- Collagen implants, made of absorbable collagen that provide temporary occlusion of the lacrimal drainage system for approximately 2 weeks duration. The implants are inserted into the canaliculi using fine tipped forceps after instilling topical anesthetic drops.
- 5-0 plain catgut suture can be used for temporary occlusion of the lacrimal drainage system for a duration of 1 to 2 weeks. The suture is cut into 3.0 mm pieces and inserted into the canaliculi using fine tipped forceps after instilling topical anesthetic drops.

Permanent Occlusion

- Silicone implants/plugs are available in different size diameters to suit the size of the lacrimal punctum. Herrick lacrimal plugs are available in 0.3, 0.5 and 0.7 mm diameter sizes. The procedure is performed on an outpatient basis, with the patient seated on the slit lamp under topical anesthesia. The punctal plug is introduced into the canaliculus, using the metal rod onto which the silicone plug is preloaded.
- Punctal cautery is performed using electrocautery or diathermy. The eyelid adjacent to the punctum is infiltrated with xylocaine 2 percent, and topical anesthetic is instilled into the cul-de-sac. The tip of the probe is threaded into the punctum and the canaliculus. The cautery or diathermy unit is switched on and blanching of the conjunctiva indicates adequate cauterization. It is important to realize that in many patients, dry eye may be due to secondary factors (systemic medications, environmental condition etc) and thus may have a waxing and waning course. A hasty decision to occlude all the four puncta permanently can lead to the development of epiphora.

Practical Pearl

The decision to occlude permanently should be made when there is evidence of presence of moderate to severe decrease in tear production with evidence of significant ocular surface disease.

PACHYMETRY

Indicated in cases corneal thickening like physiological, congenital hereditary endothelial dystrophy (CHED), corneal decompensation, scars and in case of corneal thinning like physiological, ectactic diseases like keratoconus post-traumatic. And also pre- and post-operative work up for corneal and refractive surgery.

PROCEDURE

- Turn on the unit by pressing the front panel power switch. The pachymeter will automatically perform the probe quality test and display the appropriate message indicating the quality of the probe. A probe of satisfactory quality will yield probe quality factor of 85 to 100 percent (PQF = 85-100%)
- The patient should be comfortably seated under topical anesthesia a fixation target is presented at a distance on the wall
- The probe tip is now placed on the cornea, the moment the probe is applanated a measurement is initiated
- Once a valid measurement has been obtained and the probe removed from the cornea, the pachymeter will wait for a programmed delay time before automatically storing the current measurement and advancing to the next measurement position
- Measurements are taken for superior, inferior, nasal and temporal cornea
- An average of three readings is taken for each
- A short double beep is sounded to inform the operator that the advancement has occurred
- If poor applanation occurs the machine will display a message "POOR APL"

- If either after a valid measurement or poor applanation the probe is not removed from the cornea, the pachymeter will initiate a repeat measurement after a 1.0 second delay. Only the last measurement performed is retained
- All measurements can be reviewed using the from panel switch marked or
- All measurements will remain in memory until the clear switch is pressed which will clear all measurements from memory and reinitialize the pachymeter for a measurement at position 1.

Biased measurement display: The biased data is clinically useful to the user who is taking corneal thickness measurements prior to performing refractive surgery. The surgeon may desire to set the incision depth to a predetermined bias of the actual measurement. This bias may vary as a function of the surgeon, or the knife or blade type used during the surgery.

Display Message

- *CHK PRBE:* This message usually means that the tip of the probe is wet. However, if drying the tip of the probe fails to produce an acceptable probe quality, this message may indicate that the probe has degraded and will require replacement
- *NO PRBE:* This message occurs when (1) the probe BNC connector is not mated or is improperly mated to the probe connector on the front panel or (2) The probe is defective
- *PQT FAIL:* This message usually indicates hardware failure occurred within the unit and the unit must be retuned for repair.

SPECULAR MICROSCOPY

Indications

- Corneal guttata
- Endothelial dystrophy (Fuch's)

- Prior to any surgical procedure in case of endothelial compromise
- Serial counts are taken to assess progress of corneal decompensation.

Definition of Terms

- *CD:* Cell density
- *6A:* Percentage of hexagonality
- *CV:* Coefficient of variance
- *NUM:* Number of cells taken for calculation
- *SD:* Standard deviation
- *INP:* Input.

Procedure

As soon as the patients file is obtained the following data are entered in the register.

- S.No.
- Date
- Name
- Age/Sex
- Eye
- MRD No
- Consultant
- Diagnosis
- Paying/Academic.

The patient should be comfortably seated and positioned on a adjustable chin rest. The patient is instructed to look at the fixation light (a green light). Pressing the record button snaps the picture of the corneal endothelium by autofocus and the endothelial cells are displayed. The focusing has to be changed sometimes if the picture is not displayed. To get the count of the endothelium the cells are selected by clicking it in the centre with the mouse. A minimum of 100 cells should be selected for calculation of the values and any abnormality of the cells are then entered in the file.

INFECTIVE CONJUNCTIVITIS

- Preferable to examine the patient at the earliest
- Relevant history and vision to be recorded
- Refraction, contact tonometry and dilatation of pupils can be deferred at presentation.

GRADING OF CONJUNCTIVITIS

- *Hyperacute:* Severe lid edema, chemosis and purulent discharge seen within 24 to 48 hours onset.
- *Acute:* Conjunctivitis less than 2 weeks duration.
- *Chronic:* Conjunctivitis more than 2 weeks duration.

Common causes

Hyperacute	Acute	Chronic Conjunctivitis
• Gonococcus	• Staphylococcus and other bacteria • Viral	• Chlamydia

HISTORY

- Onset and duration
- Symptoms—redness, irritation, watering and discharge (unilateral/bilateral)
- Contact with a patient with similar infection
- Recurrence.

EXAMINATION

Examine the uninvolved eye first, in case of unilateral conjunctivitis:

- *Discharge:* Quantity, color and nature
- Lid edema
- Conjunctival conjunction
- Presence of blepharitis, papillae and follicles
- Corneal evaluation
- Anterior segment examination
- Preauricular lymphnodes

- Examine the anterior segment of both eyes
- If unilateral, take care not to transfer infection to unaffected eye.

Clinical Characteristics of Bacterial Conjunctivitis

- Papillary reaction
- Mucoid or mucopurulent discharge
- Occasionally, presence of membranous conjunctivitis.

Clinical Characteristics of Viral Conjunctivitis

- Follicular reaction
- Watery, mucoid discharge
- Preauricular lymphadenopathy
- Bilateral infection (can be unilateral also).

DIFFERENTIAL DIAGNOSIS

It is important to distinguish from other common causes of red eye including allergic conjunctivitis, keratitis, nasolacrimal duct (NLD) obstruction, uveitis, acute angle closure glaucoma and episcleritis.

MANAGEMENT

- Advise ocular hygiene and stress on the contagious nature of the disease
- *Acute conjunctivitis:*
  - Bacterial conjunctivitis—patient can be started on one standard broad-spectrum topical antibiotic (e.g. Norflox or Ciplox eye drops)—frequency depending on severity of the disease
    - Viral conjunctivitis—symptomatic treatment with lubricants and weaker antibiotic like 10 percent Albucid eye drops 4 times a day
    - Review the patient periodically based on the severity
    - Instruct patient to come on an emergency basis if any worsening occurs.
- Hyperacute conjunctivitis—refer to cornea clinic.

IN THE CORNEA CLINIC

- *Conjunctival swab is advised in case of:*
  - Recent postoperative patient
  - Eyes with filtering blebs
  - Eyes with scleral buckle
  - Hyperacute conjunctivitis
  - Ophthalmia neonatorum.
- *Conjunctival scraping is advised in case of*—chronic conjunctivitis (especially to rule out *Chlamydia*).

MANAGEMENT

- Hyperacute and chronic conjunctivitis treated with topical antibiotic based on microbiological sensitivity.
- *Ophthalmia neonatorum:*
  - Elicit history of genital infection in the parents
  - Admit the patient
  - Conjunctival swab (smear report to be reviewed immediately)
  - Hourly topical antibiotic round the clock (eye drops fortified cephazoline or penicillin in case of gonococcal infection)
  - Regular cleaning of the discharge
  - Pediatrician opinion for systemic infection.

CORNEAL FOREIGN BODY

SLIT-LAMP EXAMINATION

- Meticulous examination of eye and adnexa even if corneal foreign body (FB) is visible. There may be other FBs in the conjunctival fornices, tarsal conjunctiva etc., which could be missed unless looked for
- Transparent FB may be difficult to locate in the cornea. Sclerotic scatter or retro-illumination will often highlight the presence of such FB
- Assessment of depth of FB is better done with a narrow slit and high magnification
- Look for signs of surrounding infection
- Siedel's test may be performed if a large FB is impacted in the cornea and a through–and–through perforation is suspected
- Look for evidence of an intraocular foreign body especially if there are signs of corneal or scleral perforations.

MANAGEMENT

- Superficial FBs may be removed in the general OP. A sterile cotton swab or 30G needle may be used to gently remove the FB under topical anesthesia. Instill a drop of antibiotic (e.g. tobramycin or Norflox eyedrops). If the area of epithelial defect is more than 1 mm, the eye may be patched. The patient must be reviewed the next morning to ensure healing of the epithelial defect
- In case of ferrous foreign bodies, care must be taken to remove the rust that often surrounds it
- If the FB is impacted, or if associated with signs of infection, refer the patient to cornea department.

In the Cornea Department

- If the impacted FB is know to be an inert material, e.g. glass and if it is embedded in the stroma

without signs of infection or inflammation, it may be left alone
- If the impacted FB is a large one and impaction is deep, it is best removed in the operation theatre with all sterile precautions
- If the FB is associated with infection, the FB should be sent for microbiology analysis.

OCULAR ALLERGY–ALLERGIC CONJUNCTIVITIS

INCIDENCE

Ocular allergy is growing worldwide and millions of people are affected by that, with the majority of them experiencing seasonal or perennial allergic conjunctivitis.

GLOBAL PREVALENCE

It prevails in around 15 to 20 percent of population globally.

TYPES OF ALLERGIC CONJUNCTIVITIS

Generally divided into two groups:
1. IgE dependent mast cell disease, is a class I allergic condition:
   - Seasonal allergic conjunctivitis (SAC)
   - Perennial allergic conjunctivitis (PAC)
       Mast cell sensitization due to allergen and IgE receptor activation leads to cross linking between two IgE receptors of the mast cells. This reaction leads to degranulation of mast cells with floods of histamine of the ocular surface.
2. More complex mechanism of allergic reaction involving eosinophils.
   - Vernal keratoconjunctivitis (VKC)
   - Adult keratoconjunctivitis (AKC)
   - Giant papillary conjunctivitis (GPC).

SYMPTOMS

- Ocular/periocular itching
- Redness
- Tearing
- Burning
- Stinging
- Photophobia

- Watery discharge
- Ecchymosis "allergic shiner"
- Exacerbations and remissions
- May be associated with allergic rhinitis
- May also be related to topical medications or contact lens wear.

Specific Features

- *SAC:* Occurs or reccurs at a certain period of year (summer)
- *PAC:* Manifests through out the year
- *VKC:* Occurs in childhood
- *AKC:* Occurs in adulthood
- *GPC:* Associated with contact lens wear (intolerance, awareness of lens wear or excessive lens movement are noted).

EXAMINATION

This conditions is mostly diagnosed clinically, so detailed slit lamp examinations to look for signs of allergy and rule out simulating other causes of disease become important.

- *Face and skin:* Look for allergic rashes, ichthyosis, butterfly facial rash
- *Eyelids:*
  - Look for lid edema, mucoid discharge at lid margins
  - Rule out meibomitis, blepharitis, pityriasis palpebralis.
- *Conjunctiva:* Commonly diffuse congestion of bulbar conjunctiva noted, also look for chemosis, follicular reaction, upper tarsal papillary reaction (GPC).
- *Limbus:* Papillae (VKC), Horner Trantas dots (VKC)
- *Cornea:* Superficial punctuate keratitis, Shields ulcer (VKC).

Tools for Diagnosing Allergy

- Check the patients signs and symptoms
- Proceed with thorough clinical exam

- Discuss the patient's history
- Determine if the symptom of itching is present
- Use Schirmer's test, prick test or provocation test
- Conduct a tear and conjunctival cytology(in challenging cases)
- Test of IgE intears and tear break-up time
- Collaborate with an allergist.

TREATMENT

General Measures

- Avoid rubbing eyes as it can cause mechanical degranulation of mast cells, and also touching the eye can increase the allergen load to the eye
- Washing the face, hands, changing clothes, brushing hair after reaching home from outside will definitely reduce allergen dose
- Shower before bed, so that no pollen is carried on to pillow.

Mild Cases

General measures + topical mast cell stabilizers and tear substitutes.

Moderate Cases

Above mentioned + mild steroids for 2 to 3 months.

Severe Cases

Above mentioned + higher steroids like prednisolone acetate or betnesol.

Surgical Treatment

Reserved for very severe cases includes intralesional steroids or surgical excision done for giant papillae. In recalcitrant shield ulcer debridement is done.

COMPLICATIONS

Complications are very rare with corneal ulcers or keratoconus occurring rarely.

PRACTICAL PEARLS

- Identification of the allergen by the patients should be encouraged
- Prevention is always better than cure in case of allergic conjunctivitis
- Early diagnosis and treatment may prevent complications
- Judicious use of steroids is often helpful.

VERNAL CATARRH/ALLERGIC CONJUNCTIVITIS

HISTORY

- Itching
- Mucoid discharge
- Seasonal variation
- Recurrent episodes
- *Systemic allergy:*
  - Asthma
  - Skin disease
- Drug usage (especially steroids).

EXAMINATION

- Lid edema and discoloration
- Upper lid papillae (Cobble stone papillae in vernal)
- Mucoid discharge
- Conjunctival pigmentation
- Limbal scarring (pseudogerontoxon)
- Superficial limbal keratitis
- Shield ulcer
- *Associated features:*
  - Blue sclera
  - Keratoconus.
- Cataract/glaucoma due to prolonged steroid use.

Note: Conjunctival scraping may be required to rule out other causes of follicular conjunctivitis, e.g. *Chlamydia,* virus.

MANAGEMENT

- In mild cases topical mast cell inhibitors (e.g. Cromal eye drops) for a couple of months along with tear substitutes will do
- *Counseling is extremely important with respect to:*
  - Explaining the nature of the disease
  - Use of sun glasses and cold compresses

- Need to avoid dust and pollen as much as possible
- Control of other systemic allergic conditions (asthma or skin disease if any)
- Adverse effects of long-term steroid use.

• *In moderate cases:* Mast cell inhibitor (Lodoxamide) + tapering doses of FML eye drops over a period of 1 to 2 months
• In severe or recalcitrant cases: Mast cell inhibitors + topical steroids (Betnesol or Prednisolone acetate)

Note: In case of severe papillary or follicular reaction or Shield ulcer refer to cornea department.

IN THE CORNEA CLINIC

• Tapering doses of FML eye drops over a period of 1 to 2 months in moderate to severe cases.
• Stronger topical steroid (Betnesol or Predforte) for very severe recalcitrant cases.

EXPOSURE KERATOPATHY

HISTORY

- Facial palsy
- Nocturnal lagophthalmos.

EXAMINATION

- External examination should include features of facial palsy, peri-orbital contractures and proptosis.
- Punctate keratopathy/corneal epithelial defects/ corneal ulcer/corneal vascularization involving the inferior cornea.

MANAGEMENT

- In mild cases with only minimal epithelial roughening or minimal vascularization, lubricants and nocturnal taping of the eyelids will suffice.
- Corneal ulcer to be treated as per regular protocol. Temporary or permanent tarsorrhaphy to be advised in severe cases.
- Once corneal conditions heals, oculoplasty opinion regarding lateral canthal sling procedure can be sought.

GIANT PAPILLARY CONJUNCTIVITIS

DEFINITION

- A noninfectious inflammatory disorder
- Presence of "giant" papillae (1.0 mm or greater in diameter) along the upper tarsal surface.
- Papillae measuring 0.3 mm or greater are now considered abnormal and a feature of this condition.

HISTORY

- Contact lens use–hydrophilic CL (Soft CL), rigid gas-permeable CL (RGP CL)
- *Ocular surgery:*
  - Glaucoma filtering blebs
  - Exposed sutures
  - Ocular prosthetics
  - Extruded scleral buckles.

SYMPTOMS

- Irritation
- Mucoid discharge
- Itching
- Foreign body sensation
- Reduced tolerance to CL wear
- Blurred vision with CL, increased movement of the CL.

SIGNS

- Hyperemia of the upper tarsal conjunctiva
- Conjunctival thickening
- Ropy, whitish, mucoid discharge
- Enlargement of tarsal conjunctival papillae (ranging from 0.6–1.75 mm).

MANAGEMENT

To reduce and eventually eliminate the symptoms, i.e. burning, itching, and mucus production.

- Removal of inciting agent ocular prosthesis, contact lens, exposed suture or scleral buckle
- Change of contact lens – new pair/disposable CL
- *Existing CL appears normal, then:*
  - Use preservative free solutions
  - Regular enzyme treatment of CL
  - Avoid heat disinfection of CL.
- *Pharmacologic treatment:*
  - Limited role
  - Corticosteroids, only in the acute stage to control inflammation
  - NSAIDs, questionable role
  - tear substitutes can be tried for relief of foreign body sensation
  - Mastcell stabilizers, e.g. Cromolyn sodium 4 times a day for 2 weeks.

When to Advice Patients to Resume CL Wear?
- Usually after the resolution of symptoms, when the papillae are reducing and discharge of mucus and tarsal inflammation have cleared completely
- A period of several months is usually required before restarting soft CL wear. An alternative is to fit with RGP lens
- After several years the papillae become smaller and whitish scars develop on the tops of the larger papillae.

BAND-SHAPED KERATOPATHY

HISTORY

- Duration and severity of symptoms
- Symptoms – Decreased vision, FB sensation, ocular irritation, occasional history of redness
- History suggestive of chronic uveitis
- Any Systemic disease causing hypercalcemia
- Use of topical steroid phosphate preparations, pilocarpine containing mercurial based preservatives
- Silicone oil injection in the eye
- Exposure to mercury/calcium bicarbonate vapor
- Joint pains
- Vitamin D intake
- Long standing glaucoma.

EXAMINATION

- Slit-lamp examination to look for band-shaped whitish gray, plaque like deposition across the cornea, epithelial defects and other signs of chronic uveitis, silicone oil in AC
- Look for evidence of end stage glaucoma
- Get serum Ca/serum phosphate levels
- Serum PTH levels
- Get RFT (renal function tests) done
- If suspecting sarcoidosis get serum ACE and chest X-ray done.

MANAGEMENT

- If BSK is minimal and limited to the periphery and vision is well maintained—try to treat the underlying systemic condition/cause
- To avoid excessive vitamin D intake
- If BSK is progressive despite your systemic treatment/is severe, well involving the centre of the cornea and accounting for considerable dimness of vision—refer to the cornea department.

In the Cornea Department

- Counter check history and other clinical findings
- Check Visual acuity and see if loss of vision is in proportion to the amount of corneal opacity.
- Look for associated systemic/ophthalmic findings.
- Start the treatment for underlying systemic condition if any, after reviewing the lab test reports.
- If severe BSK involving center of cornea then consider surgical debridement with 1 percent EDTA application in OT followed either by BCL insertion or by PTK with an excimer laser to smoothen the surface preferably in the same sitting.

PTERYGIUM

INTRODUCTION

A pterygium is an elevated, superficial, external ocular mass that usually forms over the perilimbal conjunctiva and extends onto the corneal surface. Pterygia can vary from small, atrophic quiescent lesions to large, aggressive, rapidly growing fibrovascular lesions that can distort the cornea, in advanced cases, they can obscure the optical center of the cornea.

HISTORY

- Irritation
- Redness
- Watering
- Dryness
- Diplopia
- Astigmatism
- Obstructed vision

CLINICAL FEATURES

A pterygium can present as any of a range of fibrovascular changes on the surface of the conjunctiva and the cornea. It is more common for the pterygium to present on the nasal conjunctiva and to extend onto the nasal cornea, although it can present temporally, as well as in other locations.

- One group of patients with pterygium can present with minimal proliferation and a relatively atrophic appearance. The pterygia in this group tend to be flatter and slow growing and have a relatively lower incidence of recurrence following excision.
- The second group presents with a history of rapid growth and a significant elevated fibrovascular component. The pterygia in this group have a more aggressive clinical course and a higher rate of recurrence following excision.

INVESTIGATIONS

- Keratometry should be done and repeated in serial follow-up periods for assessing progression, doubling of mires/difficulty in focusing as seen in advance cases.
- Corneal topography can be very useful in determining the degree of irregular astigmatism induced by advanced pterygia.
- Slit-lamp assessment and measurements of extension and external photography can assist the ophthalmologist in following the progression of the pterygium.

TREATMENT

Medical Care

Medical therapy of pterygia consists of artificial tears/topical lubricating drops and/or bland, nonpreserved ointments as well as occasional short-term use of topical corticosteroid anti-inflammatory drops when it is inflammed and symptoms are more intense. In addition, the use of ultraviolet-blocking sunglasses is advisable to reduce the exposure to further ultraviolet radiation.

Surgical Care

- Multiple different procedures have been advocated in the treatment of pterygia. These procedures range from simple excision to sliding flaps of conjunctiva with and without adjunctive external beta radiation therapy and/or use of topical chemotherapeutic agents, such as mitomycin C.
- Using free grafts of conjunctiva (with or without limbal tissue) at the same time as primary excision of the lesion has been widely advocated as the preferred treatment modality for aggressive pterygia. For moderate-to-severe pterygia, amniotic membrane can also be transplanted. Both the conjunctival autografts and the amniotic membrane

transplants may be sutured onto adjacent conjunctiva and subjacent cornea. Currently most of the surgeons seal the graft tissue onto the underlying sclera with the aid of fibrin tissue glue rather than with sutures.

Complications

- *Postoperative complications of pterygium repair can include the following:*
  - Infection
  - Reaction to suture material
  - Diplopia
  - Conjunctival graft dehiscence
  - Corneal scarring
  - Rare complications may include perforation of the globe, vitreous hemorrhage, or retinal detachment.
- *Late postoperative complications of beta radiation of pterygia can include the following:*
  - Scleral and/or corneal thinning or ectasia can present years or even decades after treatment.
  - Some of these cases can be quite difficult to manage.
- In some cases, adjunctive use of topical mitomycin-C at and after pterygium surgery has been reported to cause similar ectasia or melting of the sclera and/or the cornea.
- The most common complication of pterygium surgery is postoperative recurrence. Simple surgical excision has a high recurrence rate of approximately 50 to 80 percent. The rate of recurrence has been reduced to approximately 5 to 15 percent with use of conjunctival/limbal autografts or amniotic membrane transplants at the time of excision.
- On rare occasion, malignant degeneration of epithelial tissue overlying an existing pterygium can occur.

Prognosis

The visual and cosmetic prognosis following excision of pterygia is good. The procedures are well tolerated by patients, and, aside from some discomfort in the first few postoperative days, most patients are able to resume full activity within 48 hours of their surgery. Those patients who develop recurrent pterygia can be retreated with repeat surgical excision and grafting, with conjunctival/limbal autografts or amniotic membrane transplants in selected patients.

PRACTICAL PEARLS

- Patients should be informed about the chance of recurrence
- The surgeon should check all biopsy results after excision of pterygium to rule out the possibility of an atypical presentation of a malignancy masquerading as a benign pterygium.

CORNEAL INFECTIONS

Corneal infections (bacterial/viral/fungal rarely occur in normal eye because of eyes natural resistance to infection in the form of lids, blinking action, tears , presence of tight junction of corneal epithelium. If and when these natural defense mechanisms are breached the patient may develop keratitis (corneal infection).

RISK FACTORS

Risk factors that predispose patients to keratitis are:
- Contact lens use
- Trauma
- Previous surgery
- Immunosuppression
- Anesthesia abuse
- Ocular surface disease
- Neurotrophic keratopathy
- Systemic conditions like diabetes.

EXAMINATION

- Visual acuity
- Adnexal examination
- *Slit-lamp biomicroscopy:*
  - Circum corneal congestions
  - Presence of infiltrate—edge, activity, depth, etc.
  - Percentage of corneal thinning
  - AC reaction, hypopyon
  - Status of vitreous cavity, retina and adjacent sclera.

INVESTIGATIONS

- Smear for Grams, potassium hydroxide (KOH), and other stains if required
- Culture for bacteria and fungi
- Corneal biopsy with trephine or suture for deep infiltrates.

TREATMENT

- Topical antibiotics hourly, accordingly to culture sensitivity or broad spectrum antibiotic if culture negative for bacterial keratitis
- Topical natamycin and amphotercin B hourly for fungal keratitis
- Topical acyclovir eyedrop 5 times a day for viral keratitis. Systemic acyclovir to be included for keratouveitis
- Lubricants, antigluacoma medication and cycloplegics as applicable
- In cases of nonresolution with medical treatment, poor patient cooperation for follow-up treatment for surgical treatment in the form of therapeutic penetrating keratoplasty.

CORNEAL OPACITY

- The cornea is a transparent watchglass like structure in front of the the eyes.
- Its transparency enables the light to pass through it and form an image onto the retina.
- Any opacity of the cornea can lead to a drop in vision.

CONDITIONS THAT CAUSE CORNEAL OPACITY
0 to 5 Years Age
Mnemonic for the causes of congenital clouding of the cornea: STUMPED
- *S:* Sclerocornea
- *T:* Tears in the Descemet's membrane secondary to birth trauma or congenital glaucoma
- *U:* Ulcers
- *M:* Metabolic
- *P:* Peters anomaly
- *E:* Edema (CHED)
- *D:* Dermoid

5 to 35 Years Age
- Epithelial/stromal dystrophy
- Hydrops
- Interstitial keratitis
- Crocodile shagreen
- Nummular opacity
- Ulcer.

>35 Years Age
- Fuchs endothelial dystrophy
- Aphakic/pseudophakic bullous keratopathy
- Band-shaped keratopathy
- Arcus senilis
- Spheroidal degeneration
- Ulcer.

APPROACH TO A PATIENT WITH CORNEAL OPACITY

History

- *Onset:* The opacity if present from birth/or acquired–this history is of utmost importance when discussing the prognosis of the vision in the eye as an opacity from child could be associated with underlying amblyopia. These patients must, therefore, be forewarned of the possibility of low visual potential even if the treatment/surgical procedure goes well
- *History of trauma:* If so the details of it to assess the status of the lens/any retained foreign body in presence of traumatic cataract— important in visual potential of the eye
- *History of associated pain, redness, watering, discharge:* Associated with aphakic/pseudophakic bullous keratopathy, viral endothelits, interstitial keratitis, ulcer/abscess, hydrops
- *History of past surgery:* Posterior segment, intraocular lens (IOL) implantation—eyes that have undergone repeated retinal detachment (RD) surgeries with silicone oil are more prone to develop band shape keratopathy
- *History of associated refractive error/frequent change of glass prescription in the past:* This can be suggestive of a previous keratoconus that may present as a hydrops
- *History of associated cough, cold, fever:* Presenting with discharge/nummular lesions—indicate viral etiology
- *History of associated systemic problems:* Hyperlipidemia, hypercalcemia can be associated with lipid keratopathy/band-shape keratopathy in an otherwise virgin eye.

CLINICAL FEATURES

- *Visual acuity:* To be documented and correlated with the corneal opacity so as not to miss associated

lens changes/retinal lesions that may be contributory.
- *Location:* Of the opacity with respect to the pupil (visual axis) and with respect to the layers involved (bowman's, anterior stromal, posterior stromal, Descemet's membrane)
  - A faint small lesion in the visual axis is more troublesome than a dense lesion in the periphery of the cornea
  - Its location must be documented as ....mm from the limbus/in clock hours involved.

Size of The Lesion

It is to be documented as it may be useful in planning graft size for surgery.
- *Density of the lesion:* (nebular, macular , leucoma)
- *Laterality:* Bilateral conditions are usually dystrophy/degenerations
- *Associated vascularity/ghost vessels (how many clock hour involvement):* It is important to determine the prognosis of the graft as extensive vascularity > 2 clock hours can increase the chances of rejection
- *Status of the limbus:* Since a limbal insufficiency can give rise to problems in epithelialization post-operatively
- Associated thinning of the cornea
- Associated pigmentation.
- Lid closure, status of tear function—for maintenence of the graft
- *IOP:* Must be brought under contol prior to surgery and maintained for the survival of the graft.

TREATMENT

- Any acute condition needs treatment first—like hydrops, interstitial keratitis, viral endothelitis Visual rehabilitation can be sought for after the eye has quietened down
- Small corneal opacity not in visual axis can be left alone

- *Contact lens:* Contact lens can be used for small, nebular opacity in visual axis, corneal irregularity caused by scar. Rigid gas permeable (RGP) lenses are used
- *Corneal transplant:* Penetrating keratoplasty, deep anterior lamellar keratoplasty (DALK), Descemet's stripping endothelial keratoplasty (DSEK) can be planned depending on depth of involvement, compliance of patient
- In addition amniotic membrane transplantation (AMT), limbal transplantation may be done in patients with vascularization
- Amblyopia therapy in children.

DERMOID

INTRODUCTION

Dermoid and epidermoid cysts are examples of choristomas, tumors that originate from aberrant primordial tissue. These tumors contain normal-appearing tissue in an abnormal location. They may contain a variety of histologically aberrant tissues, including epidermal appendages, connective tissue, skin, fat, sweat gland, lacrimal gland, muscle, teeth, cartilage, bone, vascular structures, and neurologic tissue, including the brain. Malignant degeneration is extremely rare.

HISTORY

- Dermoids are present at birth but may not be recognized until the first or second decade of life
- They may also appear to enlarge as the body matures
- Growth of these lesions is generally slow
- Occasionally, a history of inflammation will be present
- In limbal dermoids visual morbidity may result from encroachment of the lesion into the visual axis, development of astigmatism, or formation of a lipid infiltration of the cornea.

Associated ocular abnormalities include coloboma of the eyelids, Duane retraction syndrome and other ocular motility disorders, lacrimal anomalies, scleral and corneal staphylomata, aniridia, and microphthalmia. Associated systemic abnormalities include preauricular appendages and auricular fistulae (in combination with limbal dermoids constituting Goldenhar syndrome). Other abnormalities include hemifacial microsomia, microtia, and vertebral anomalies.

CLINICAL FEATURES

- The diagnosis of a dermoid requires a directed clinical examination. Specific laboratory studies are generally not necessary
- Imaging studies may be required for orbital demoids.

TREATMENT

- Dermoid cysts usually are cosmetic problems. The location of the dermoid cyst in the orbit helps determine the appropriate type of orbitotomy. A method for percutaneous drainage and ablation of orbital dermoid cysts and endoscopic-assisted removal of orbital dermoid cysts has been reported
- Inflammation from preoperative or intraoperative rupture of the cyst can be controlled with use of steroids
- Treatment of limbal dermoids may consist of periodic removal of irritating cilia, topical lubrication to prevent foreign body sensation, or excision of the lesion if it is causing significant cosmetic disfigurement or interfering with vision
- A superficial sclerokeratectomy, cutting flush with the surface of the globe, is the procedure of choice for removal of the dermoid. Excised tissue always should be sent to the pathologist for examination
- Attempts at complete removal are unnecessary. The lesion may extend into the deeper structures of the eye and the risk of perforation increases if attempts are made to remove the lesion completely
- The exposed sclera should be covered by relaxing the adjacent conjunctiva and sewing it into the scleral defect. If a deep excision is necessary, then a lamellar keratoplasty can be performed to reinforce the site of excision
- A young patient presenting with a limbal dermoid may be at a risk of developing amblyopia. Likewise, a patient presenting with a limbal dermoid may

have already developed amblyopia. The rate of amblyopia in patients suffering from limbal dermoids has been reported to be present in up to 50 percent of the patients. This issue must be discussed with the patient and/or the patient's family.

CORNEAL ECTASIA

- The cornea is a transparent structure in front of the eyes with a normal radius of curvature ranging from 40 D to 45 D accounting for approximately 66 percent of the refractive power of the eye
- In certain conditions the curvature of the eye increases gradually and progressively and is termed as ectasia.

SYMPTOMS

- Progressive myopia—frequent change in spectacles
- Irregular astigmatism
- Ghosting of images
- Fluctuating vision
- Problems with scotopic vision (vision in darkness or dim lighting)
- Progression of ectasia leads to severe loss of–corrected visual acuity
- Eyes at high risk of corneal ectasia following LASIK may have unstable refractions and variable posterior surface bowing prior to developing frank ectasia.

CAUSES OF CORNEAL ECTASIA

- Genetic conditions like keratoconus, pellucid marginal degeneration, keratoglobus
- Postrefractive surgery ectasia
- Terriens marginal degeneration
- Posttrauma, conditions like peripheral corneal ulcer
- Children with allergic condition with constant rubbing of the eyes.

KERATOCONUS

Usually bilateral noninflammatory thinning of the cornea which leads to irregular astigmatism. Most commonly occurs in the inferotemporal quadrant, it may present as an apical cone or oval cone usually demarcated by the Fleischer's ring in advanced cases. Thinning occurs at the point of maximum protrusion.

KERATOGLOBUS

Bilateral ecstatic disorder characterized by globoid protrusion and thinning of the cornea. May occur isolated or associated with Leber's Amaurosis, blue sclera, extensible joints, hearing abnormalities.

PELLUCID MARGINAL DEGENERATION

Bilateral, inferior (rarely superior) peripheral corneal thinning characterized by a narrow band of thinning below the area of maximum protrusion, with an uninvolved area of the cornea present between the thinning and the limbus. It typically presents with a butterfly pattern in the topography.

TERRIENS MARGINAL DEGENERATION

Inflammatory cause of peripheral thinning of the cornea usually seen superiorly.

POSTREFRACTIVE SURGERY ECTASIA

Myopic refractive error with increased astigmatism, worse spectacle corrected visual acuity, increased corneal toricity with topo abnormalities, progressive corneal thinning.

APPROACH TO THE PATIENT
History

- The patient may present with any of the above symptoms, or asymptomatic with frequent change of spectacles.
- A high index of suspicion is required in the diagnosis of early stages of keratoconus, PMD.
- Associated symptoms like decreased night vision, eczema, asthma, Down's syndrome, heart abnormalities, etc. must be enquired for.

EXAMINATION

Reflexes

- *Retinoscopy:* The reflex in retinoscopy will show a split in the image called scissoring reflex because the light reflected back passes through different portions of the cornea having different refractive power.
- Indirect ophthalmoscopy shows classical Charleux oil droplet sign.

Anterior Segment Examination

- *Munson's sign* is the V shape protrusion of the lower lid in down gaze.
- *Steep cornea* can be appreciated in moderate to severe cases.
- *Vogts striae* are vertical stress marks in the descemets membrane at the apex of the cone.
- *Fleischer's ring* are iron pigment line at the base of the cone it is best appreciated in red free light.
- *Thinning of the cornea* is usually at the apex of the cone in keratoconus and blow or abow the apex in PMD.
- Scarring of the anterior stroma, Bowmans layer may be seen .

INVESTIGATIONS

- Keratometry
- Pachymetry
- Corneal topography
- Pentacam/Orbscan
  Are the parameters needed to confirm the clinical diagnosis and identify any progression of the condition.
  Corneal topography indices to be looked for are:
  - Keratometry (K) value more than 47 D
  - Interior superior dioptric assymetry (I-S) value > 1.6 D
  - KISA percent more than 100

Pachymetry an added value of pachymetry has emerged due to the new procedure called corneal collagen cross linking for stopping the progression of corneal ectasia.This procedure can be done when the ectasia has been documented to be progressing but the corneal thickness above 400 microns.

Pentacam/orbscan is useful in identifying posterior corneal changes which may be missed prior to refractive surgery.

TREATMENT

- *Medical:* Refractive correction in the form of spectacles, contact lenses (rigid CL, piggy back, rose K, scleral lenses) can be used to provide good visual outcome.
- *Surgical:* Surgical options are undertaken only as a last resort when CL becomes unbearable, and the cone has progressed extensively. Corneal transplantation PK/ DALK can be done depending upon the extent of scar formation present.
- *Newer modalities:* Corneal collagen crosslinking involves the strengthening of the cornea by creating crosslinking between the collagen fibers and there by strengthening it by instilling riboflavin eyedrops and exposing the cornea to ultraviolet rays.

CORNEAL DYSTROPHY

The term "corneal dystrophy" has been used to refer to a group of inherited corneal diseases that are typically bilateral, symmetric, slowly progressive and without relationship to environmental or systemic factors.

In clinical practice, we may find corneal dystrophy presentation to be straightforward or subtle. Patients can present with discomfort, blurred vision, or neither. It is important to make a proper diagnosis so as to properly educate patients about the genetics, prognosis, and management options.

CLASSIFICATION

The International Committee of Classification of Corneal Dystrophies (IC3D) have developed a new classification system for corneal dystrophies that utilizes the understanding of the genetics of each condition to categorize the dystrophies. These categories are as follows (Weiss et al, 2008):

Category-1: A well-defined corneal dystrophy in which a gene has been mapped and identified and specific mutations are known.

Category-2: A well-defined corneal dystrophy that has been mapped to one or more specific chromosomal loci, but the gene (or genes) remain to be identified.

Category-3: A well-defined corneal dystrophy that has not yet been mapped to a chromosomal locus.

Category-4: Reserved for suspected new or previously documented corneal dystrophies, although the evidence for such dystrophies being separate and distinct is not yet convincing.

The most commonly used method for categorizing corneal dystrophies is by the layer of tissue in which they are located. These categories can be broken down into epithelial and subepithelial dystrophies, Bowman's layer dystrophies, stromal dystrophies, and endothelial and Descemet's membrane dystrophies. Table 3.1 outlines the various dystrophies by layer with inheritance and IC3D categorization (Weiss et al, 2008).

Diagnosing Corneal Dystrophies

When attempting to diagnose a corneal dystrophy, it is important to consider the layers involved, the age of the patient, the family history, and the type of findings. Most corneal dystrophies have an early onset and are genetic, so at presentation, the parents and patient are often already aware of the familial condition.

However, in situations in which this is not the case, careful evaluation of the types of findings and their location, along with some type of resource, can help you make the proper diagnosis. Table 3.2 lists corneal dystrophies along with onset, symptoms and signs to aid in differentiating the dystrophies (Weiss et al, 2008).

Eventually, you can base your diagnosis of a corneal dystrophy potentially upon the patient's symptoms and slit lamp observation, and this can be corroborated with the patient's family history in most cases.

Managing Corneal Dystrophies

Once the diagnosis of dystrophy is made, the decision regarding management depends on the severity of symptoms. Many will have little or no ocular or visual symptoms and will thus require little or no treatment. For patients who do have symptoms, treatment options again depend on the layer of the cornea in which the disease is found and the type of symptoms the patient has.

Table 3.1: Corneal dystrophies categorized by corneal layer with inheritance and IC3D category (Weiss et al, 2008)

Dystrophy	Inheritance	IC3D category
Epithelial and subepithelial		
Epithelial basement membrane dystrophy (EBMD)	Sporadic	1 (When applicable)
Epithelial recurrent erosion dystrophy (ERED)	AD	4, 3
Subepithelial mucinous corneal dystrophy (SMCD)	AD	4
Meesmann's corneal dystrophy	AD	1
Lisch epithelial corneal dystrophy	XD	2
Gelatinous drop-like corneal dystrophy	AR	1
Bowman's layer dystrophies		
Reis-Buckler's corneal dystrophy	AD	1
Thiel-Benke corneal dystrophy	AD	2
Grayson-Wilbrandt corneal dystrophy	AD	4
Stromal dystrophies		
Lattice type 1 corneal dystrophy	AD	1
Granular corneal dystrophy	AD	1
Macular corneal dystrophy	AR	1
Schnyder corneal dystrophy	AD	1
Congenital stromal corneal dystrophy	AD	1
Fleck corneal dystrophy	AD	1
Posterior amorphous corneal dystrophy	AD	3
Central cloudy dystrophy of Francois	Unknown	4
Pre-Descemet's corneal dystrophy	Unknown	4
Descemet's membrane and endothelial dystrophies		
Fuchs' endothelial corneal dystrophy, late onset	Unknown, some AD	2
Fuchs' endothelial corneal dystrophy, early onset	AD	1
Posterior polymorphous corneal dystrophy 1	AD	2
Posterior polymorphous corneal dystrophy 2	AD	1
Posterior polymorphous corneal dystrophy 3	AD	1
Congenital hereditary endothelial dystrophy 1	AD	2
X-linked endothelial corneal dystrophy	XS	2

Table 3.2: Corneal dystrophies with onset, symptoms and signs to aid in differentiating and diagnosis (Weiss et al, 2008)

Dystrophy	Figure	Onset	Symptoms	Signs
Epithelial and subepithelial				
Epithelial basement membrane dystrophy (EBMD)	1	Adult	Corneal erosions, mild visual reduction	Areas of thickened epithelium, round or oval opacities, lines
Epithelial recurrent erosion dystrophy (ERED)	2	1st decade of life	Painful erosions, burning, redness, photophobia	None, other than when erosions are present
Subepithelial mucinous corneal dystrophy (SMCD)	3	1st decade of life	Painful recurrent erosions	Bilateral subepithelial opacities and haze
Meesmann's corneal dystrophy (Stocker-Holt variant) Symptoms more severe in Stocker-Holt variant	4	Early childhood	Mild corneal erosions, some visual reduction	
Lisch epithelial corneal dystrophy	5	Childhood	Asymptomatic or blurred vision if visual axis is affected	Localized gray opacities in various shapes: whorls, bands, flames, or feather shaped

Contd...

Contd...

Dystrophy	Figure	Onset	Symptoms	Signs
Gelatinous drop-like corneal dystrophy	6	1st to 2nd decade	Decreased vision, photophobia, irritation, redness, tearing	Subepithelial lesions in bands or clusters that exhibit late staining, superficial vascularization is common
Bowman's layer dystrophies				
Reis-Buckler's corneal dystrophy	7	Childhood	Visual impairment, painful recurrent erosions	Confluent irregular opacities at the level of Bowman's membrane and superficial stroma
Thiel-Benke corneal dystrophy	8	Childhood	Painful recurrent erosions with gradual visual impairment	Subepithelial reticular (honeycomb) opacities mainly in the central cornea. Can progress fully into stroma
Grayson-Wilbrandt corneal dystrophy	—	1st to 2nd decade	Mild visual reduction and mild recurrent erosions	Diffuse mottling/grayish opacities at Bowman's membrane that extend anteriorly into epithelium. Stroma may have refractile opacities
Stromal dystrophies				
Lattice type 1 corneal dystrophy Lattice type 2 (less severe, later onset, (+) systemic signs)	9, 10	1st decade	Discomfort, pain, and visual impairment, recurrent erosions	Thin, branching, refractile lines and/or subepithelial dots at onset, ground glass haze develops later

Contd...

Contd...

Dystrophy	Figure	Onset	Symptoms	Signs
Granular corneal dystrophy types 1 and 2	11, 12	Childhood	Glare, photophobia, recurrent erosions possible	Well-defined white opacities that appear as confluent granules. Type 2 can add snowflakes and lattice lines between granules
Macular corneal dystrophy	13	Childhood	Severe visual reduction, photophobia, painful recurrent erosions possible	Limbus-to-limbus stromal haze initially, later superficial, central, elevated white opacities
Schnyder corneal dystrophy	14, 15	Childhood to 3rd decade	Visual acuity decreases with age, glare increases	Initial signs include central haze and subepithelial crystals (up to age 23), Arcus lipoides between age 23 and 38, midperipheral panstromal haze after age 38
Congenital stromal corneal dystrophy	16	Congenital	Moderate to severe vision loss	Diffuse, bilateral corneal clouding with flake-like whitish opacities distributed throughout the cornea. Increased corneal thickness with pachymetry
Fleck corneal dystrophy	17	Congenital	Asymptomatic	Small, translucent, disc-shaped opacities or gray-white flaky opacities with clear stroma in between

Contd...

Contd...

Dystrophy	Figure	Onset	Symptoms	Signs
Posterior amorphous corneal dystrophy	18	1st decade possibly congenital	Mild visual reduction	Diffuse gray-white, sheet-like opacities mainly in the posterior stroma. Corneal thinning and flat topography are often present. Many other minor signs possible
Central cloudy dystrophy of Francois	19	1st decade	Mostly asymptomatic	Cloudy central polygonal or rounded stromal opacities
Pre-Descemet's corneal dystrophy	20	1st decade to adult	Asymptomatic	Focal, fine gray opacities in deep stroma, some lesions can be larger, shapes vary greatly
Descemet's membrane and endothelial dystrophies				
Fuchs' endothelial corneal dystrophy, late onset	21	5th decade or later	Intermittent reduced vision; when severe, burst epithelial bullae can cause pain	Corneal guttata (generally larger) and stromal edema
Fuchs' endothelial corneal dystrophy, early onset	—	1st decade or later	Intermittent reduced vision, when severe burst epithelial bullae can cause pain	Corneal guttata (generally smaller) and stromal edema

Contd...

Contd...

Dystrophy	Figure	Onset	Symptoms	Signs
Posterior polymorphous corneal dystrophy types 1, 2 and 3	22	Early childhood	Generally asymptomatic, rarely visual reduction may occur	Deep lesions, may have nodular, vesicular, and/or blister-like shapes. Railroad track appearance. Rarely stromal and epithelial edema occur with corresponding complications
Congenital hereditary endothelial dystrophy type 1	23	1st or 2nd year of life	Blurred vision, photophobia, and tearing	Minimal signs, cornea diffusely hazy or milky with or without gray spots
Congenital hereditary endothelial dystrophy type 2	—	Congenital	Blurred vision, often nystagmus	Same as type 1 but more severe
X-linked endothelial corneal dystrophy (males)	24	Congenital	Blurred vision, possible nystagmus	Clouding, haze, ground glass appearance. May have moon crater-like endothelial changes
X-linked endothelial corneal dystrophy (females)	—	Congenital	Asymptomatic	Moon crater endothelial changes only

Medical Treatment of Corneal Dystrophies

1. Topical medications are often a first line of therapy for many conditions-lubricants. In patients who have corneal dystrophies and experience ocular discomfort that is mild.
2. Antibiotic drops may be required during episodes of erosions that are significant enough to warrant coverage.
3. Topical steroids can be used in situations in which chronic photophobia, redness, and watering are issues, provided that you monitor the patient for potential side effects.
4. Hyperosmotic agents may also benefit patients who have corneal dystrophies that have resulted in corneal edema.

Contact Lens Treatment of Corneal Dystrophies

Contact lenses can have a wide spectrum of application for corneal dystrophy patients, from
- Soft lenses for recurrent erosions to
- GP lenses for visual rehabilitation to
- Scleral lenses for both of these reasons.

Surgical Management of Corneal Dystrophies

There are many options for surgical management of corneal dystrophies, and the options continue to evolve. Choosing the procedure again depends on the level of the dystrophy.

1. Epithelial debridement is a technique for treating recurrent erosions resulting from corneal dystrophy. Removing the weak, loose epithelium and allowing the epithelial cells to readhere to the basement membrane seems to reduce recurrences to about 20 percent.
2. Anterior Stromal Puncture (ASP) for recurrent erosions is based on the theory that the resultant scarring causes better epithelial adhesion.

3. Phototherapeutic Keratectomy (PTK), is a more common approach to treating recurrent erosions. PTK is a safe and effective way to reduce recurrences of erosions and to improve acuity in some cases, although a hyperopic shift should be assumed and accounted for in advance.

4. Keratoplasty is an option for treating corneal dystrophies when symptoms are severe enough to warrant the procedure. In the past, full thickness grafts were the only good option. However, with the advent of more useful lamellar procedures, corneal transplants can be an option earlier in the course of treatment for some. Since many corneal dystrophies are confined mainly to specific layers of the cornea, a lamellar graft can be successfully utilized for some dystrophy patients.

4a. Deep anterior lamellar keratoplasty (DALK) is a lamellar graft that involves removing the epithelium, Bowman's layer, and as much of the stroma as possible, while leaving the endothelium and Descemet's membrane intact and can be useful for anterior dystrophies, the primary advantage being a reduced risk of rejection.

4b. Posterior lamellar grafts utilized in endothelial layer dystrophies are mainly Descemet's stripping automated endothelial keratoplasty (DSAEK) and Descemet's membrane endothelial keratoplasty (DMEK).

   – DSAEK involves removing the diseased endothelium and Descemet's membrane by simply stripping it manually and replacing it with donor tissue, which consists of endothelium, Descemet's membrane, and a thin layer of stroma. The donor tissue is prepared by use of an automated keratome.

   – DMEK procedure removes the diseased tissue the same way, but strips the same tissue off of the donor graft manually. By not transplanting any stromal tissue, the visual outcomes are improved; however, the complexity of the procedure is greater and the risk of graft slippage is higher at this stage of its evolution.

Full thickness penetrating keratoplasty is an option for corneal dystrophy patients when a lamellar graft is not indicated.

Recurrence of dystrophic findings in corneal transplants is common, with rates reported at approximately 70 percent for any findings and 15 to 20 percent at five years for clinically significant findings including recurrent erosions and loss of vision.

Managing corneal dystrophies can be difficult. As the condition continues to deteriorate and is no longer amenable to management by conservative measures, surgical options can be utilized with generally good results, though recurrences should be anticipated.

CORNEAL GRAFT REJECTION

PRESENTING SYMPTOMS

- Decreased vision
- Pain
- Redness
- Photophobia.

HISTORY

- Time of surgery
- Visual recovery after surgery
- Surgical details
- History of previous episodes
- Current medications/Recent change of medications
- Previous ocular disease leading to penetrating keratoplasty PK.

EXAMINATION

- Check visual acuity
- *Slit-lamp examination—look for critical signs of graft rejection:*
  - Graft clarity—edema, infiltrates.
  - Subepithelial infiltrates or epithelial line.
  - New keratic precipitates on endothelium.
  - Presence of loose sutures.
  - Presence of vascularization.
  - Any synechiae at host-graft junction.
  - Intraocular pressure.

If any of the above critical signs are present refer to Cornea Department.

At the Cornea Clinic
- Document symptoms and signs
- Categorize (Epithelial/Subepithelial/Endothelial)·

MANAGEMENT

- Topical steroids (Predforte 1%) 1 hourly while awake.
- Topical antibiotics (Ciplox) 6 to 8 times a day

- Cycloplegic agent – homatropine 2 to 3 times per day
- If rejection is less than one week admit the patient and start IV methylprednisolone 500 mg over 30 minutes period after obtaining clearance from the physician
- Systemic steroids 40 to 80 mg PO once a day with Tab Rantac (150 mg) or Syp Gelusil (monitor BP, blood glucose, weight gain)
- Control intraocular pressure if raised (topical Timolol 0.5 percent bid if patient is not an asthmatic and has no cardiac problem)
- Antivirals topical acyclovir and Tab acyclovir 250 mg five times daily is to be given if the PK was done for postviral etiology
- *In case of high risk PKs—immunosuppression high-risk PK:*
  - Highly vascular corneas
  - Regrafts
  - Only eye
  - Previous rejection episodes
  - Extensive synechiae.

IMMUNOSUPPRESSION

Imuran—1 mg/kg/day
- Monitor complete blood counts and platelets. Stop if platelet count is less than 1 lakh/cmm or white blood cells (WBC) count is less than 5000/cmm

Cyclosporin—for prevention and treatment of rejection 2.5 mg/kg/day.
- Monitor for nephrotoxicity—serum creatinine every 2 weeks. BP every visit, hepatotoxicity (liver function tests).

Follow-up

- Every 3 to 7 days
  - Once there is improvement, gradual tapering of steroids and maintain low doses for several months
  - Intraocular pressure check must be done regularly.

OCULAR SURFACE DISEASE

Ocular surface disorders can vary in manifestation ranging from mild dryness related discomfort to corneal blindness secondary to end stage conditions like, chemical injuries, Stevens Johnson syndrome and ocular cicatricial pemphigoid. A thorough evaluation and tailored approach is mandatory to diagnose the condition and consider varied available management options. Most of these are chronic conditions that can be controlled but rarely cured.

BROAD CLASSIFICATION

1. Dysfunctional tear syndrome
   - Dry eye with lid margin disease
   - Dry eye without lid margin disease
   - Tear distribution anomalies (conjunctivochalasis).
2. Cicatricial conjunctival disorders
   - Mucus membrane pemphigoid
   - Stevens Johnson syndrome
3. Chemical injuries
4. Limbal stem cell deficiency–primary/secondary
5. Others.

DYSFUNCTIONAL TEAR SYNDROME

Dry Eye

National Eye Institute Definition

"A disorder of the tear film due to tear deficiency or excessive evaporation, which causes damage to the interpalpebral ocular surface and is associated with symptoms of ocular discomfort ".

This definition is more clinically oriented with not much emphasis on the pathogenetic mechanisms or the events that occur in response to dry eye.

DEWS Definition

"Dry eye is a multifactorial disease of the tears and ocular surface that results in symptoms of discomfort, visual disturbance, and tear film instability with potential damage to the ocular surface. It is accompanied by increased osmolarity of the tear film and inflammation of the ocular surface."

The International Dry Eye WorkShop (DEWS) have developed a 3-part classification of dry eye, based on:
- Etiology (aqueous deficiency/evaporative state)
- Mechanisms (osmolarity and instability) and
- Disease stage (Table 3.3).

Delphi Panel Suggestion

The term dry eye does not reflect all the events occurring in the eye and hence recommended *dysfunctional tear syndrome (DTS)* as a more appropriate term for this disease. However, the term dry eye is so embedded in medical literature and lay writing, that the term DTS has been replaced by *dry eye disease*.

DIAGNOSTIC TESTS

History Taking

History taking forms an integral part of the ocular examination in dry eye and often helps in revealing associated conditions that could aggravate the ocular problem. Most types of dry eye are more common in women, especially post menopausal. Diseases with a poor prognosis such as Stevens-Johnson syndrome associated tear dysfunction usually have an abrupt onset of signs and symptoms. Leading questions help ascertain if the condition has progressed since inception or not. Dry eye states with an underlying immune disorder generally tend to progress relentlessly, while others such as ocular cicatricial pemphigoid have a characteristic chronic recurrent pattern. Any

Table 3.3: Classification of dry eye

Dry eye severity level	1	2	3	4
Discomfort, severity and frequency	Mild and/or episodic; occurs under environmental stress	Moderate episodic or chronic, stress or no stress	Severe frequent or constant without stress	Severe and/or disabling and constant
Visual symptoms	None or episodic mild fatigue	Annoying and/or activity-limiting episodic	Annoying, chronic and/or constant, limiting activity	Constant and/or possibly disabling
Conjunctival injection	None to mild	None to mild	+/−	+/++
Conjunctival staining	None to mild	Variable	Moderate to marked	Marked
Corneal staining (severity/location)	None to mild	Variable	Marked central	Severe punctate erosions
Corneal/tear signs	None to mild	Mild debris, decreased meniscus	Filamentary keratitis, mucus clumping, increased tear debris	Filamentary keratitis, mucus clumping, increased tear debris, ulceration
Lid/meibomian glands	MGD variably present	MGD variably present	Frequent	Trichiasis, keratinization, symblepharon
TFBUT (sec)	Variable	≤10	≤5	Immediate
Schirmer score (mm/5 min)	Variable	≤10	≤5	≤2

treatment that the patient has received in the past should be noted as also the perceived response of the patient to the prescribed medications.

History taking should include:

a. Patient Symptoms
b. Occupational and Medical History
c. Associated Systemic Disorders
d. Importance of Rapport Building.

CLINICAL TESTS

Tear Secretion Assessment

Schirmer's Test

Schirmer's 1: < 5 mm at 5 minutes is considered abnormal.

Schirmer's 2: It is performed as above along with nasal stimulation using a cotton tipped applicator. A value of < 10 mm at 5 minutes is considered abnormal.

Abnormality in both tests is indicative of lacrimal gland dysfunction affecting both the normal and reflex tear secretion.

Schirmer's 3: It was originally described similar to Schirmer's 1 along with retinal stimulation by looking at the sun and is no longer performed.

Jones basal tear secretion: It is performed similar to Schirmer's 1 but with application of anesthetic drop prior to placement of the strips.

Tear Volume Assessment

Tear meniscus height: The lower meniscus is examined for its height, regularity, width and curvature. The normal tear meniscus height is 0.1 to 0.3 mm.

Tear Clearance Assessment

Tear clearance test: The fluorescein clearance test (FCT) is a dynamic tear functional test to reveal basic tearing, reflex tearing and tear clearance simultaneously. FCT is performed as follows:

After applying one drop of 0.5 percent proparacaine to each eye, the inferior fornix is carefully dried with tissue paper. An aliquot of 5 µl of fluorescein 0.25 percent (if not available, dye impregnated strips can be used) is applied in the inferior conjunctival cul-de-sac without directly touching the conjunctival surface. The patient is asked to blink normally. Schirmer's testing is carried out for 1 minute at the end of 10, 20 and 30 minutes respectively. At the end of the 30 minutes, i.e. the last test, Schirmer strip is inserted after nasal stimulation with cotton tipped applicator. Clearance is defined as normal if the dye cannot be detected at the 20-minute interval.

The FCT allows one to determine the following three important tear dynamic functions, i.e. basal tear secretion, reflex tear secretion under nasal stimulation, and tear clearance at the same time.

Its clinical applications are:
1. To determine aqueous tear deficiency (dry eye) with higher accuracy.
2. To differentiate dry eye into with or without reflex tearing. Sjogren syndrome or primary lacrimal gland diseases are characterized by the loss of reflex tearing, thus helping establish the severity of dry eye.
3. To guide physicians to perform punctal occlusion with plugs or permanent cauterization.
4. To determine subclinical DTC as a cause of ocular irritation, medicamentosa and other ocular surface disorders.

FLUOROPHOTOMETRY

Tear Function Index (TFI)

Evaluation of Tear Film Stability

Tear break-up time

An unstable tear film is the hallmark of dry eye. Invasive and noninvasive techniques are available to assess the stability. A value of > 10 seconds is considered normal for both TBUT and NIBUT, reflects tear film instability, whereas less than 5 seconds is a marker of definite dry eye.

Lipid Layer Assessment
Meibomian Gland Dysfunction

Biomicroscopic recognition of pathological signs such as ductal orifice metaplasia (white shafts of thickened meibum in the orifices), reduced expressibility of meibomain gland secretions, increased turbidity and viscosity of the expressed secretions and dropout of glandular acini aids in diagnosis of MGD.

Ocular Surface Damage Assessment
Diagnostic Dye Staining

The use of dyes such as fluoroscein, rose-bengal, and lissamine green helps in assessing the
* Integrity of the ocular surface epithelium
* Protective status of the precorneal tear film.

Impression Cytology

It has been useful in the investigation of many aspects of dry eye disease such as
* Pathophysiology of dry eye (degree of squamous metaplasia)
* Monitoring clinical trials (to evaluate efficacy of treatments)
* Associating dry eye disease with other systemic conditions.

Tear Osmolarity

In patients with dry eye the impaired balance between tear secretion, evaporation and clearance leads to an increase in tear osmolarity, which is considered one of the major sources of discomfort, ocular surface damage and inflammation.

Its cut-off value is 315.6 mOsm/L between healthy and dry eyes.

Tear Protein Assays

Corneal sensitivity: In routine clinical practice a cotton wick can be used to assess the presence or absence of corneal sensation.

MANAGEMENT

The foremost objectives in caring for patients with dry eye disease are to improve the patient's ocular comfort and quality of life, and to return the ocular surface and tear film to the normal homeostatic state. Although symptoms can rarely be eliminated, they can often be improved, leading to an improvement in the quality of life.

Avoidance of Exacerbating Factors

Environmental modifications such as:
– Humidification
– Avoidance of wind or drafts, and
– Avoidance of dusty or smoky environments may ameliorate dry eye symptoms.

Lifestyle or workplace modifications may be helpful, for example,
– Taking regular breaks from reading or computer use
– Lowering the computer monitor below eye level so that the gaze is directed downward.
– Increasing blink frequency or fast blinking exercises have also been recommended.

If feasible, medications that exacerbate disease should be discontinued.

Eyelid Hygiene

Tear supplementation: Ocular lubricants or artificial tear are mainstay of dry eye treatment.

Tear Retention

1. Punctal occlusion—punctal plugs or Punctal cautery.
2. Moisture chamber spectacles.
3. Tarsorrhaphy.

Tear stimulation: Secretagogues

Several potential topical pharmacologic agents may stimulate aqueous secretion, mucous secretion, or both. The agents currently under investigation are diquafosol (one of the P2y2 receptor agonists), rebamipide, gefarnate, ecabet sodium (mucous secretion stimulants), and 15(S)-HETE (MUC1 stimulant).

Two orally administered cholinergic agonists, pilocarpine and cevilemine, have been evaluated in clinical trials and found to be marginally beneficial.

Biological Tear Substitutes

1. Autologous serum tears.
2. Autologous platelet rich plasma.
3. Salivary gland autotransplantation.

Anti-inflammatory Therapy

1. Topical cyclosporin.
2. Corticosteroids.
3. Oral tetracyclines.
4. Essential omega-3 fatty acids.

Treatment of underlying systemic condition, if any: The International Dry Eye Work Shop (DEWS) Subcommittee members reviewed the Delphi Panel (the Dry Eye Preferred Practice Patterns of the American Academy of Ophthalmology and the International Task Force Delphi Panel on Dry Eye) approach to the treatment of dry eye and modified it. Treatment recommendations are based on disease severity.

- *Level 1:*
  - Education and environmental/dietary modifications
  - Elimination of offending systemic medications
  - Preserved artificial tear substitutes, gels, and ointments
  - Eyelid therapy (for MGD)·

- *Level 2:* If level 1 treatment is inadequate, add the following:
  - Nonpreserved artificial tear substitutes
  - Anti-inflammatory agents
    - Topical corticosteroids
    - Topical cyclosporine A
    - Topical/systemic omega-3 fatty acids
  - Tetracyclines (for MGD)
  - Punctal plugs (after control of inflammation)
  - Secretagogues
  - Moisture chamber spectacles
- *Level 3:* If level 2 treatment is inadequate, add the following:
  - Autologous serum
  - Contact lenses
  - Permanent punctal occlusion
- *Level 4:* If level 3 treatment is inadequate, add the following:
  - Systemic anti-inflammatory agents
  - Surgery
    - Lid surgery
    - Tarsorrhaphy
    - Mucous membrane grafting
    - Salivary gland duct transposition
    - Amniotic membrane transplantation.

CHEMICAL INJURIES

Etiology

Chemical injuries to the eye can result in mild injury, or severe ocular damage. Mostly victims are young and exposure occurs in workplace particularly in an industrial setting, at home, and in association with criminal assaults. Most chemical injuries are due to acid or alkali compounds, with the latter being more common.

The extent of ocular involvement depends on several factors:

- The strength of the chemical agent,
- Concentration,

- Volume of solution, and
- Duration of exposure.

Pathophysiology

In general, alkalis tend to penetrate more effectively than acids.

Alkalis result in:
- Saponification and disruption of fatty acids in cell membranes, leading to cell death
- Hydration of glycosaminoglycans results in loss of clarity of the stroma
- Elevation in intraocular pressure
- Intraocular structures may also be affected
- Stromal corneal ulceration.

In acid injuries the hydrogen ion causes damage due to pH alteration, while the anion produces protein precipitation and denaturation in the corneal epithelium and superficial stroma producing the ground glass appearance of the epithelium. This barrier may protect against weaker acids, but strong acids may continue to penetrate deeply.

Classification

A useful classification of chemical injuries was first proposed by Hughes and then modified by Roper-Hall (Table 3.4). This classification divides the clinical manifestations into four categories which help to guide prognosis and treatment. This classification has become the commonly used benchmark since its introduction in 1965.

Dua et al proposed a significant modification to the Roper-Hall classification to take into account the extent of limbal involvement in clock hours, and the percentage of conjunctival involvement (Table 3.5). Clock hours of the limbus were determined by dividing the limbus into 12 hours of a clock face. It was concluded that with present management strategies like autolimbal or allolimbal transplantation, with or without amniotic membrane transplantation, an eye

Table 3.4: Classification of severity of ocular surface burns by Roper-Hall

Grade	Prognosis	Cornea	Conjunctiva/ Limbus
I	Good	Corneal epithelial damage	No limbal ischemia
II	Good	Corneal haze, iris details visible	<1/3 limbal ischemia
III	Guarded	Total epithelial loss, stromal haze, iris details obscured	1/3–1/2 limbal ischemia
IV	Poor	Cornea opaque, iris and pupil obscured	>1/2 limbal ischemia

Table 3.5: New classification of ocular surface burns

Grade	Prognosis	Clinical findings	Conjunctival involvement	Analog scale*
I	Very good	0 clock hours of limbal involvement	0%	0/0%
II	Good	Up to 3 clock hours of limbal involvement	Up to 30%	0.1–3/ 1–29.9%
III	Good	>3–6 clock hours of limbal involvement	>30–50%	3.1–6/ 31–50%
IV	Good to guarded	>6–9 clock hours of limbal involvement	>50–75%	6.1–9/ 51–75%
V	Guarded to poor	>9–<12 clock hours of limbal involvement	>75–<100%	9.1–11.9/ 75.1–99.9%
VI	Very poor	Total limbus (12 clock hours) involved	Total conjunctiva (100%) involved	12/100%

*The analog scale records accurately the limbal involvement in clock hours of affected limbus/percentage of conjunctival involvement. While calculating percentage of conjunctival involvement, only involvement of bulbar conjunctiva, up to and including the conjunctival fornices is considered.

with 50 percent or even 75 percent limbal ischemia can expect a good to fair outcome, whereas an eye with 100 percent ischemia is very likely to have a poor outcome.

TREATMENT

Treatment can be divided into acute and chronic management strategies. Acute treatment is primarily medical, and chronic management may require surgical therapy. Management of chemical injury must attempt to:

1. Promote ocular surface epithelial recovery
2. Augment corneal repair
3. Control inflammation.

Treatment in the Acute Phase of Injury

Chemical injuries constitute a true ophthalmic emergency and immediate ocular irrigation is necessary prior to taking history, or completing the rest of the ocular exam.

1. An isotonic solution with a neutral pH is preferable, such as normal saline or Ringer's lactate, any nontoxic solution is acceptable in an emergency. Irrigation should continue for a minimum of thirty minutes, or until the pH becomes neutral.
2. Debridement of the necrotic corneal tissue.
3. A broad-spectrum topical antibiotic such as ciprofloxacin would be prudent to avoid a microbial keratitis.
4. Frequent lubrication with preservative free eye drops should be utilized to enhance epithelialization.
5. Bandage soft contact lenses with careful follow-up.
6. Topical corticosteroids can be utilized to decrease inflammation in the first 7 to 10 days of treatment
7. Topical NSAIDs such as ketoralac.
8. Sodium ascorbate 10 percent hourly or 1000 mg of oral ascorbic acid four times.
9. Tetracycline and its derivatives may be added for anticollagenolytic effect.
10. Sodium citrate 10 percent hourly.

11. A glass rod can be used to break developing symblepharon on a daily basis and helps to prevent shortening of fornices. Alternatively a symblepharon ring can be used with a bandage contact lens.
12. Tissue adhesives like cyanoacrylate glue are effective tool for management of impending or actual perforation related to sterile ulceration of the corneal stroma following chemical injury.

Surgical Management in Acute Phase

1. *AMT:* For large nonhealing epithelial defects, amniotic membrane transplantation (AMT) can be performed in the acute stage.
2. *Tenonplasty:* It is recommended in cases of persistent scleral and limbal ischemia in combination with amniotic membrane transplantation.
3. *Tectonic graft:* It is performed in case of large corneal perforation.

Management in Chronic Phase

Prior to undertaking any visual rehabilitative procedures, it is extremely important to correct any associated glaucoma through medical and/or surgical means and address surface inflammation. Fornix reconstruction forms the initial phase of rehabilitation in order to stabilize the tear film and better the success of subsequent limbal transplantation.

Limbal Stem Cell Transplantation

In unilateral chemical injuries with total limbal stem cell deficiency, the procedure of choice would conjunctival limbal autograft (CLAU).
It is usually performed in a staged manner:
• Fornix reconstruction
• Limbal autograft (CLAU or exvivo limbal stem cell transplant)
• Lamellar or penetrating keratoplasty for corneal opacity.

In bilateral chemical injuries, limbal allograft can be performed. However, this procedure is associated with a high risk of rejection and requires long-term immunosuppression.

Keratoprosthesis may be useful for bilateral, severe chemical injury where the prognosis is hopeless for penetrating keratoplasty due to irreparable damage to the ocular surface or repeated immunological rejection.

1. Boston KPro has established its role in restoring vision to patients suffering from corneal blindness from various pathologies including chemical injuries. Overall, the Boston KPro is capable of restoring media clarity and demonstrates good anatomic retention. But patients with chemical burns are a more difficult group to manage due to presence of concomitant preoperative ocular disease, particularly glaucoma and high extrusion rates.

2. Modified osteo-odonto-keratoprosthesis that uses the autologous tooth as a carrier for the polymethylmethacrylate is reserved for the more severe cases of chemical injury. It has shown to provide long-term, anatomically stable corneal prosthesis as well as an effective rehabilitating recovery in visual acuity.

STEVENS-JOHNSON SYNDROME

Stevens-Johnson syndrome (SJS), though an acute self limited disorder of the skin and mucus membrane, leads to chronic cicatricial changes in the eye. In the acute stage of the disorder, much attention is given to the life threatening systemic disturbances, thus neglecting the ocular involvement. The ocular manifestations in the acute stage include ocular inflammation and tarsal ulceration, including corneal complications in a few cases. This further goes on to incite scarring and subsequent cicatrisation leading to the chronic ocular sequelae of SJS. Though self limited, we are aware of the chronic continuing episodes of inflammation in SJS.

Management of Ocular Condition in the Acute Stage

1. Copious lubrication
2. Broad spectrum antibiotics
3. Topical steroids, if necessary
4. Monitor epithelial healing
5. Amniotic membrane transplantation (lid margin to lid margin) has been shown to be beneficial, if performed within the first 2 weeks of onset of SJS.

Causes for Persistent Inflammation in SJS

1. Dry eye
2. Lid margin keratinization
3. Adnexal disorders—trichiasis, distichiasis, entropion
4. Conjunctival inflammation secondary to underlying pathophysiology.

Differential Diagnosis

It has to differentiated from ocular cicatricial pemphigoid (OCP) in cases where history is not definitely suggestive of SJS especially in the elderly. OCP has to be monitored for evidence of progression in subsequent visits. It has to managed along with an immunologist. Dapsone usually is recommended in early stages and cyclophosphamide in the advanced cases of OCP to control inflammation.

Management in Chronic Stage

1. *Management of dry eye:*
   - Copious lubrication
   - Punctal occlusion(cautery)
2. Correction of trichiasis, entropion
3. *Lid margin keratinization:*
   - Boston scleral lens
   - Mucous membrane grafting

4. *Anti-inflammatory:*
   - Preservative free topical steroids in cases of persistent inflammation following correction of dry eye and other mechanical causes of inflammation
   - Systemic immunosuppression may be required in some cases with severe persistent inflammation
5. *Visual rehabilitative procedures:*
   - Boston scleral lens in case of corneal irregularity
   - *In case of cataract:* Cataract extraction after addressing all of the above
   - *Keratoprosthesis:* Modified osteo-odonto kerato-prosthesis (MOOKP) is the procedure of choice in end-stage SJS and OCP with surface keratinization.

OCULAR SURFACE SQUAMOUS NEOPLASIA

Tumors of the stratified squamous epithelium of the conjunctiva and cornea encompasses a wide spectrum of lesions, ranging from benign disturbances of epithelium maturation (actinic keratosis, pseudo epitheliomatous hyperplasia) to frank malignant neoplasia (squamous cell carcinoma and its variants).

HISTORY AND PREDISPOSING FACTORS

Patients can present as with:
- Conjunctival mass
- Irritation and foreign body sensation
- Redness.

Common systemic predisposing factors include:
- Exposure to ultraviolet light
- HIV positivity
- Xeroderma pigmentosa
- HPV.

EXAMINATION

Most lesions are located in the bulbar conjunctiva, at the limbus and are often gelatinous appearance with papillomatous surface. Size of the tumor, presence of leukoplakia, feeder vessels, mobility, preauricular and submandibular lymph nodes should be noted.

Detailed drawing of the tumor site, size and color is an essential prerequisite in the working of a patient with ocular surface squamous neoplasia.

INVESTIGATIONS

- Rose Bengal staining to delineate the tumor extent
- Impression cytology in doubtful cases
- Gonioscopy, UBM to detect depth of the tumor
- CT scan and MRI to determine orbital involvement
- HIV screening.

MANAGEMENT

- Surgical excision is the treatment of choice in localized tumor. Excision of the lesion with a safe margin of 2 to 3 mm is often adequate. Cryotherapy to the limbus and conjunctival margins reduces the recurrence rate. Specimen should be sent for histopathological diagnosis. Extensive lesion with orbital involvement requires exentration.
- Medical management includes topical cytotoxic agents (mitomycin C, 5-fluorouracil) has been used to debulk extensive tumors before surgery or to treat small early recurrences.

PRACTICAL PEARLS

- Careful history and preoperative evaluation
- Meticulous surgery with no touch technique is mandatory to minimize recurrences
- Periodic postoperative review to detect recurrences.

4

Glaucoma

- Primary Open Angle Glaucoma
- Guidelines for Target Intraocular Pressure
- Other Commonly seen Glaucomas and Related Conditions
- Classification of Medications and Adverse Events
- OPD Procedures

PRIMARY OPEN ANGLE GLAUCOMA

HISTORY

- Symptoms—ocular pain, headache, vision loss, field defects, haloes
- Onset, progress from previous records
- Positive family history—details of disease, outcome and surgery
- Baseline intraocular pressure (IOP), maximum IOP, diurnal profile if available
- Medications if any—list of drugs currently in use, allergies, response pattern, time of last application of medications
- Management details
  - Argon laser trabeculoplasty—details
  - Surgery—details
- Systemic illness—especially bronchial asthma

EXAMINATION

- Best corrected visual acuity
- Ocular alignment and motility
- Pupil reactivity and function (important in asymmetric disease)
- *Slit-lamp examination:*
  - Pre- and postdilatation examination
    - Pseudoexfoliation glaucoma
    - Coexisting cataract
  - Signs of secondary glaucoma
  - Corneal edema
  - Pigment on the posterior surface of the cornea and anterior chamber (AC)
  - AC reaction and keratic precipitates
  - Iris—color, contours, defects, pupillary ruff defects, transillumination defects, iris atrophy, neovascularization
  - Exfoliation flakes

- Shape and thickness of crystalline lens, marks of previous trauma are signs of secondary glaucoma
- *Intraocular pressure (Applanation tonometry):*
  - Note time and last application of medications
  - Diurnal variation as and when needed
- Gonioscopy—to be done at least once a year or once in 6 months after use of miotics
- Indirect ophthalmoscopy
- *Stereo examination with biomicroscopy of the disc (78 or 90 D):*
  - Size and shape of disc and cup, cup disc ratio (CDR), nerve fiber layer defects
  - Site of thinning, peripapillary atrophy—type, location and extent
  - Site of disc hemorrhage.

INVESTIGATIONS

- Visual field examination
- A must in diagnosis and follow up. Minimum of two field examinations are generally needed for baseline evaluation. Dilatation is done for miotic pupils or lens changes if significant.
  - *Central 30-2 SITA:* Standard usually
  - *SITA-fast or Stimulus Size V:* If visual acuity is low or poor cooperation on the part of patient is expected
  - *Central 10-2:* In advanced disease with tunnel fields
  - *Macular threshold:* Before surgery to assess for postoperative outcome and for assessing macular wipeout phenomenon.
- Disc photography (stereo)—in selected patients
- Short wavelength automated perimetry (SWAP), GDx nerve fiber analyzer and optical coherence tomography (OCT)—in selected patients
- Pachymetry (ultrasonic)—for evaluating central corneal thickness in selected patients (Ref: OHT study)

GENERAL CRITERIA FOR DIAGNOSIS

- IOP > 21 mm of Hg
- Open angles
- Cupping > 0.3:1 CDR with typical nevroretinal rim NRR changes
- Visual field changes corresponding to disc changes fulfilling Anderson's criteria (Ref: Anderson and Patella – Automated perimetry).

MANAGEMENT

- Patient education - regarding glaucoma and side effects of therapy
- Institute therapy (choice of medication depends on patient's disease condition, amount of IOP reduction needed, patient's financial status, compliance, age and systemic status)
  - *Topical medication:*
    - ◆ Single medication with less side effects
    - ◆ Unilateral trial and adequate follow-up
    - ◆ Explain lid closure and nasolacrimal duct (NLD) blockage after medication
    - ◆ Ensure compliance each time
    - ◆ Switch over therapy to better drugs than addition
  - *Surgery:*
    - ◆ If maximal tolerable medical therapy (MTMT) fails
    - ◆ An extremely noncompliant patient
  - *Argon laser trabeculoplasty:*
    - ◆ Patients with MTMT but who refuse surgery
    - ◆ Noncompliant patients until surgery.
- Mild exercise, avoiding stress and control of systemic illnesses are advised
- Inform regarding risk to other family members and importance of screening. If positive family history exists, patient is referred for genetic counseling and blood analysis.

GUIDELINES FOR TARGET INTRAOCULAR PRESSURE

Minimum of 20 percent reduction from baseline IOP is required as target IOP to prevent progression

Initial average IOP (mm Hg)

Visual field loss	50	40	30	20
Mild	30	25	23	16
Moderate	25	25	20	14
Severe	20	20	15	10

FOLLOW-UP

- Ensure compliance and ask for adverse events with drugs
- Maintenance of disc drawings, descriptions
- Follow-up visual field examinations – depends on disease severity which is assessed by IOP control and disc changes:
  - If stable, field testing once a year
  - If unstable, 2 months to 6 monthly evaluation
  - If a new disc hemorrhage is seen, visual fields is done immediately and two months later to look for progression. Disc hemorrhage may need aggressive management
  - Confirm progression before advising change of medications or especially surgery by repeating visual fields
- Reset target IOP if progression is present in spite of reaching the previously fixed target IOP and institute therapy accordingly.

Guidelines for follow-up (Ref: PPP of AAO 1999)

Target IOP reached	Progression of damage	Duration of control (in months)	Follow-up
Yes	No	Less than 6	1 to 6 months
Yes	No	More than 6	3 to 12 months
Yes	Yes	Not applicable	1 week to 3 months
No	No	Not applicable	1 day to 3 months
No	Yes	Not applicable	1 day to 1 month

Note: Always remember that the disease is chronic and will not lead to blindness in a few months. At the same time one must understand that certain patients progress inevitably to blindness in spite of aggressive management.

OTHER COMMONLY SEEN GLAUCOMAS AND RELATED CONDITIONS

Diagnosis and follow-up mostly are like primary open angle glaucoma (POAG). Variations are given below.

ACUTE ANGLE CLOSURE GLAUCOMA

Diagnostic Points

Acute onset symptoms, signs of angle closure and elevated IOP, closed angles.

Management

- Admit and initiate IV mannitol therapy along with maximum antiglaucoma and anti-inflammatory medications
- Ensure inflammation has subsided and IOP is controlled with clearing of cornea in the affected eye
- Examine the other eye for angle occludability—YAG peripheral iridotomy to both eyes. If not possible, think of surgical peripheral iridotomy (PI) or trabeculectomy.

CHRONIC ANGLE CLOSURE GLAUCOMA AND CREEPING ANGLE CLOSURE GLAUCOMA

Diagnostic Points

- Quiet eye
- Shallow anterior chamber
- Raised IOP
- Peripheral anterior synechiae on gonioscopy.

Management

- As in POAG
- Prophylactic peripheral iridotomy.

OCULAR HYPERTENSION
Diagnostic Points

Intraocular pressure more than 21 mm of Hg with otherwise normal features including visual fields.

Management

- Rule out risk factors
- Pachymetry to rule out increased central corneal thickness
- Discuss options of observation and follow-up
- Initiate treatment if IOP >28 mm of Hg generally
- SWAP, GDx and OCT may be helpful in certain patients
- Examination of family members.

NARROW OR OCCLUDABLE ANGLES
Diagnostic Points

More than 180° angle closure at least up to posterior trabecular meshwork with or without positive provocation tests (no dilatation is done before peripheral iridotomy to prevent mydriasis induced angle closure).

Management

- Prophylactic peripheral iridotomy
- Examination of family members.

CONGENITAL GLAUCOMA
Diagnostic Points

- Presence of large corneal diameter or increasing size
- Corneal changes with raised IOP (usually with tonopen)
- Increased axial length by B-scan ultrasonography
- Angle anomalies in gonioscopy (done under anesthesia)
- Cupped disc.

Management

- Explain nature and prognostic outcome to both parents:
  - Possible need for multiple procedures
  - Risk of anesthesia
  - Future possibility of corneal procedures (in selected patients)
  - Amblyopia and its management
  - Inborn errors of metabolism and TORCH done in selected patients to rule out infective and metabolic causes
- Examination under anesthesia (neonates need to get fitness from a neonatologist) combined with surgical approach.
  - Usually external trabeculectomy
  - In severe disease and relatively advanced age, trabeculectomy is needed.

Follow-up

- Examination in OPD for IOP, corneal diameter, disc changes and axial length with B-scan done once in at least a year in stable patients. If not possible, to do under anesthesia
- The same applies for post-lensectomy, post VR surgery, ROP, pediatric IOL patients seen in all the departments.

PIGMENTARY GLAUCOMA

Diagnostic Points

- Krukenberg's spindle
- Iris transillumination defects
- Dense trabecular meshwork pigmentation
- Concave iris configuration.

Management

- As for POAG
- ALT may have a role in some patients (it has better outcome compared to POAG as per ALT trial)

- Prophylactic peripheral iridotomy in selected patients after discussing the option (if irido-zonular contact is present on UBM)
- Aqueous suppressants and miotics are avoided—prostaglandins are preferred.

PSEUDOEXFOLIATION GLAUCOMA

Diagnostic Points

- Pseudoexfoliation (PXF) material on pupillary ruff, angle, corneal endothelium
- Nondilating pupil
- Typical PXF pattern on lens
- Subluxation of lens.

Note: Most often dilatation is needed for evaluating PXF.

Management

- As in POAG
- May be associated with narrow angles needing PI.
- Combined surgery – management of poorly dilating pupil and risk of subluxation
- UBM preferred in selected patients for evaluating zonules.

NORMAL TENSION GLAUCOMA

Diagnostic Points

- History of acute hypotensive episodes, migraine, peripheral vascular diseases and hematological disorders.
- IOP < 21 mm of Hg on a diurnal variation.
- Otherwise similar to POAG.
- Disc hemorrhage more frequent
- Visual fields can have deeper steeper defects closer to the fixation

Management

- As in POAG
- Record corneal thickness (may have variable thickness)

- Remember approximately 50 percent may not progress.
- Needs aggressive management if initial IOP in low teens.
- Exclude neurological and systemic vascular causes if indicated by a pale disc with typical field changes.

NEOVASCULAR GLAUCOMA

Diagnostic Points

Neovascularization (NVI), NVA, ischemic retinal features with or without neovascularization of the optic disc (NVD) or neovascularization elsewhere (NVE).

Management

- Establish cause of neovascularization
- Identify the stage of the disease
- *If blind or visual potential poor:*
  - Conservative approach in the form of symptomatic treatment
  - IOP control achieved by medications or cyclo-destructive procedures
  - In severe cases, may require enucleation with ball implant. Rarely retrobulbar alcohol injection can be tried for pain relief
- If visual potential is present and treatable retinal condition identified (CRVO, PDR): Panretinal photocoagulation with or without peripheral retinal ablation.

PLATEAU IRIS SYNDROME

Diagnostic Points

- Flat iris contour
- Incomplete opening of angles on gonioscopy, volcano crater appearance with compression
- Raised IOP with patent PI on dilatation.

Management

- UBM may be used for diagnosis
- Prophylactic peripheral iridotomy with medications (especially miotics)

- Argon laser iridoplasty in selected patients
- Surgery in uncontrolled patients.

Note: Avoid frequent dilatation – dilate only with weak cycloplegics such as tropicamide 1 percent.

PHACOMORPHIC GLAUCOMA

Diagnostic Points

- Uniformly shallow AC with centrally more shallowing
- Intumescent or hypermature cataract
- Closed angles.

Management

- Examination of other eye for occludable angle
- Control of IOP with maximum medications
- Prophylactic peripheral iridotomy for both eyes as indicated
- If less than two weeks—early cataract extraction with IOL implantation
- If more than two weeks – combined cataract surgery with trabeculectomy may be needed.
- Surgery done under mannitol cover—small incision cataract surgery may be preferred.

PHACOLYTIC GLAUCOMA

Diagnostic Points

Presence of inflammation, mature cataract, fluffy lens or milky cortical material in AC and angle.

Management

- Medical control of IOP and inflammation
- Early cataract extraction with IOL implantation
- If IOP uncontrolled with medication or long-standing problem (approximately more than 2 weeks), trabeculectomy may be needed
- Surgery done under mannitol cover if needed.

POST-TRAUMATIC GLAUCOMA
Diagnostic Points

- Inflammation
- Hyphema
- Subluxated lens
- Ghost cells in AC
- Elevated IOP
- Angle recession

Note: Avoid gonioscopy in the presence of hyphema.

Management

- Medical control of IOP and inflammation
- If IOP uncontrolled with medication, trabeculectomy may be needed
- Subluxated lens may need removal
- *Management of hyphema:*
  - Do not apply pressure over the eye
  - Rule out clotting disorders
    - Basic coagulation profile for all cases
    - Detailed coagulation profile for suspected bleeding disorders.
  - Eight ball hyphema, ghost cells in AC and corneal staining need early hyphema evacuation
  - If IOP not under control with medication, do hyphema evacuation and follow-up IOP control.

Note: In case of bleeding diathesis, the surgery is done with necessary supplements in consultation with a hematologist, e.g. factor VIII for hemophilia.

POSTINFLAMMATORY GLAUCOMA
Diagnostic Points

- *Presence of inflammation:*
  - KPs (old or fresh)
  - Steroid induced (look for depot)
  - Iris bombe
  - Iris atrophy
  - Synechial angle closure

Management

- *Elevated IOP and inflammation:* Medical control
- *Iris bombe:* Prophylactic PI under steroid cover— topical ± systemic
- *Steroid induced (if clinically appears short term):*
  - Medical control of IOP for 2 months after cessation of all steroids
  - Then discontinued and re-evaluate IOP
  - If IOP elevates again—resume medical control or surgery
  - Patient explained the chances of POAG later in life.
- IOP to be monitored at least yearly and lifelong
- Periodic IOP and gonioscopy is a must in chronic uveitis to document angle features.

PUPILLARY BLOCK GLAUCOMA

Diagnostic Points

- Inflammatory synechiae
- Silicone oil or gas in posterior chamber
- Subluxated normal or microspherophakic lens.

Management

- Medical control of IOP and inflammation
- *Pupillary block with silicone oil – order of management options:*
  - Prophylactic YAG PI
  - Surgical PI
  - SOR with or without filtering surgery or endocyclophotocoagulation depending on visual potential and available conjunctiva for filter. Valve implants advised in selected patients
- *Subluxated and microspherophakic lens (steps in management):*
  - Try repositioning lens in supine position
  - Pilocarpine eyedrops with or without IV mannitol
  - Prophylactic PI

- Advise lensectomy with or without scleral fixated IOL if recurrence is anticipated. Filtering surgery with antimetabolites needed in case of associated glaucoma.

IRIDOCORNEAL ENDOTHELIAL SYNDROME

Diagnostic Points

- Middle-aged female
- Iris and/or corneal changes, iris adhesions on gonioscopy.

Management

- Specular microscopy and pachymetry
- Medical control of IOP
- Usually needs surgery with antimetabolites
- Refractory to treatment.

NANOPHTHALMOS

Diagnostic Points

- Small palpebral fissure
- High hyperopia
- Very shallow AC
- Normal lens with small ocular parameters on A-scan, axial length < 19 mm.

Management

- A-scan for AC depth, lens thickness, axial length
- PI if needed
- Control of IOP and follow-up as routine
- Explain the need for careful cataract surgery with or without filtering surgery
- Use of prophylactic sclerotomies in all cases during any intraocular procedure.

ELEVATED EPISCLERAL VENOUS PRESSURE-INDUCED GLAUCOMA

Diagnostic Points

- Raised IOP with dilated episcleral vessels
- Blood in Schlemm's canal with gonioscopy.

Management

- B-scan for superior ophthalmic vein
- Rule out fistulas (MRI preferable)
- Rule out systemic disease like hypo- or hyper-thyroidism and other causes of elevated episcleral venous pressure
- Treat systemic condition
- Control IOP medically—if not amenable, trabeculectomy with antimetabolites.

MALIGNANT GLAUCOMA

Diagnostic Points

- Shallow or flat AC
- Patent PI
- Elevated IOP in postsurgical situation
- Anteriorly rotated ciliary processes on UBM in the absence of other causes.

Management

- UBM for above findings (If choroidal effusion present, conservative approach may help)
- *Medical control:*
  - Antiglaucoma medications especially aqueous suppressants including systemic acetazolamide
  - Cycloplegics (need to be continued for a minimum of 6 months to lifelong)
  - Steroids during acute phase
- YAG hyaloidotomy in pseudophakes and aphakes
- Vitrectomy (with or without lensectomy) in selected situations.

CLASSIFICATION OF MEDICATIONS AND ADVERSE EVENTS

Table 4.1: Beta-adrenergic antagonist

Class	Generic name	Trade name	Concentrations	Dosing regimen	Major side effects	Mechanism(s) of IOP reduction
Nonselective β_1/β_2-adrenergic antagonists	Timolol maleate	Glucomol Nyolol	0.25%, 0.5%	Two times a day	Bradycardia Bronchospasm Fatigue Impotence Hypotension	Decreases aqueous humor production
	Timolol maleate gel forming solution	Timolet GFS Timoptic XE	0.25%, 0.5%	One time a day		
	Levobunolol hydrochloride	Betagan	0.25%, 0.5%	One-two times a day		
	Carteolol hydrochloride	Ocupress	1%	One-two times a day		
	Timolol hemihydrate	Betimol	0.5%	One-two times a day		
Selective β_1-adrenergic antagonist	Betaxolol hydrochloride	Optipress	0.5%	Two times a day	Bradycardia Bronchospasm Fatigue	Decreases aqueous humor production
	Betaxolol hydrochloride suspension	Betoptic–S Optipress	0.25%	Two times a day		

Table 4.2: Nonselective adrenergic antagonist

Class	Generic name	Trade name	Con-centrations	Dosing regimen	Major side effects	Mechanism(s) of IOP reduction
Nonselective α- and β -adrenergic agonists	1. Dipivefrin hydrochloride		0.1%	Two times a day	Allergy Conjunctival hyperemia	Increases traditional outflow facility
	2. Epinephrine hydrochloride	Epifrin	0.5%, 1% 2%	Two times a day	Cystoid macular edema Headache	
	3. Epinephrine borate	Epinal	0.5 – 1%	Two times a day	Hypertension Tachycardia Mydriasis	

Table 4.3: Selective α_2^- adrenergic agonist

Class	Generic name	Trade name	Con-centrations	Dosing regimen	Major Side effects	Mechanism(s) of IOP reduction
Selective α_2-adrenergic agonists	Apraclonidine	Iopidine Alfa drops	0.5%, 1% 0.5%, 1%	Two times a day to three times a day Used in laser procedures	Allergic blepharo-conjunctivitis Dry mouth Fatigue	Decreases aqueous humor production
	Brimonidine	Alphagan and Alphagan P Alphagan Z	0.20% 0.15%	Two times a day	Dry mouth Fatigue Drowsiness	Decreases aqueous humor production and increases uveo-scleral outflow

Table 4.4: Carbonic anhydrase inhibitors

Class	Generic name	Trade name	Con-centrations	Dosing regimen	Major side effects	Mechanism(s) of IOP reduction
Topical carbonic anhydrase	Dorzolamide	Trusopt	2%	Two or three times a day	Bitter taste	Decreases aqueous humor production
	Brinzolamide	Azopt	1%	Two or three times a day	Blurred vision	Decreases aqueous humor production
Oral carbonic anhydrase inhibitors	Acetazolamide	Diamox	125 mg 250 mg	Four times a day	Anemias Electrolyte imbalance Fatigue	Decreases aqueous humor production
		C. Iopar S R Diamox Sequel	250 mg 500 mg	Two times a day	Gastrointestinal disturbances Kidney stones	
	Dichlorphenamide	Daranide	50 mg	Two-three times a day	Malaise Metabolic acidosis	
	Methazolamide	Glauctabs	25–50 mg	Two-three times a day	Paresthesias Polyuria Stevens-Johnson syndrome	

Table 4.5: Prostaglandin related drugs

Class	Generic name	Trade name	Con-centrations	Dosing regimen	Major side effects	Mechanism(s) of IOP reduction
Prostaglandin analog	Latanoprost	Xalatan	0.005%	Once at night	Cystoid macular edema	Increases uveoscleral outflow
Prostamides	Bimatoprost	Lumigan	0.03%	Once at night	Increased iris pigmentation	
Docosanoid derivative	Unoprostone	Rescula	0.15%	Two times a day	Eyelash lengthening and darkening uveitis	
Prostanoid agonist	Travoprost	Travatan	0.004%	Once at night		

Table 4.6: Miotics

Class	Generic name	Trade name	Con-centrations	Dosing regimen	Major side effects	Mechanism(s) of IOP reduction
Miotics	Pilocarpine	Pilocar Isoptocarpine Pilogel Locarpgel	1%, 2%, 4%	2, 3 and 4 times a day	Punctual stenosis, hypersensitivity, miosis, accommodative spasm, retinal hole, iris cyst, cataract	Increases trabecular outflow

Table 4.7: Combinations

Class	Generic name	Trade name	Dosing regimen
Combinations	Latanoprost + Timolol	Xalacom	Once a day
	Timolol +Dorzolamide	Cosopt	Twice a day
	Timolol + Brimonidine	Combigan	Twice a day
	Timolol + Pilocarpine	Timolet plus	Two to three times a day
		Timpilo	Once a day
	Timolol + Bimatoprost	Lumigan	Once a day
	Timolol + Travoprost	Travacom	Once a day

OPD PROCEDURES

Procedure	Indications	Settings	Postoperative medications	Remarks and follow-up
Nd:YAG PI	Occludable angles Acute ACG Chronic ACG Plateau iris Nanophthalmos Pupillary block glaucomas	Abraham lens 2 mJ – 6 mJ/shot Superonasal or superotemporal quadrant Minimum 150 microns opening	Tab Acetazol 1 stat; topical steroids 4–6 days	IOP check 1 hour; 1 day and 2 weeks later
ALT*	POAG PDS PXF glaucoma	Goldmann 3 mirror lens 180° or 360° 500 to 1000 mW 0.1 second Jn of pig. TM and non- pig. TM	As above Continue antiglaucoma Rx and taper	As above + monthly till IOP control seen
ALI	Plateau iris syndrome	Goldmann 3 mirror lens 180° or 360° 500 to 1000 mW 0.1 second Peripheral iris	As above Continue antiglaucoma Rx and taper	As above + monthly till IOP control seen

Contd...

Contd...

Procedure	Indications	Settings	Postoperative medications	Remarks and follow-up
Diode cyclo-photocoagulation	MTMT in all glaucomas with low visual potential and symptomatic glaucomas (if surgery is not possible)	G probe 1.5 mm from limbus 1200 – 2000 mW 2000 ms 20 to 40 shots 180° to 360°	As above Continue antiglaucoma Rx and taper	As above
Cyclocryotherapy	-do-	Retinal probe 2 mm from limbus 80°C × 1 minute/ application Freeze-thaw-freeze technique	As above Continue antiglaucoma Rx and taper	As above
5-FU injections	To reduce wound healing at the bleb site post-trabeculectomy	5 mg of 0.1 cc 5-FU in tuberculin syringe injected with 30 g needle	Postoperative steroids	Review next day
Argon laser suturelysis ALS	To lyse the suture post-trabeculectomy to control IOP	Spot 50 microns Energy 300 mJ Interval 100 ms	Nil	IOP check after 1 hour

* ALT is done only in selected patients who do not want surgery or unable to undergo surgery with MTMT and uncontrolled IOP

$$5$$

Uvea

- Anterior Uveitis
- Intermediate Uveitis
- Posterior Uveitis
- Panuveitis
- Scleritis
- Retinal Vasculitis
- Use of Steroids and Immunosuppressive Agents
- Cataract Surgery in Uveitis
- Investigations in Uveitis
- Investigations for Tuberculosis
- Interpretation of Laboratory Tests for Toxoplasmosis
- Interpretation of Laboratory Tests for Human Immunodeficiency Virus
- Interpretation of Laboratory Tests for Cytomegalovirus
- Anterior Chamber Tap
- Periocular Steroid Injection in Uveitis
- Subconjunctival Injection of Mydricaine
- Intravenous Acyclovir (Acivir or Zovirax)
- Intravitreal Ganciclovir Injection in CMV Retinitis

ANTERIOR UVEITIS

DEFINITION

Inflammation of the iris and the ciliary body is known as anterior uveitis.

POINTS TO BE NOTED DURING HISTORY TAKING

Patient Details

- Age—Juvenile rheumatoid arthritis (JRA) is common in patients less than age 15 years
- Sex—JRA is common in females, HLA– B27 associated uveitis in males.

Ocular History

- Is the disease unilateral or bilateral?
- When was the first attack?
- When was the last/current attack?
- What was the approximate frequency of the attacks between the first and the last attacks?
- Details of prior ocular treatment.
- Any previous history of rise in intraocular pressure (or use of any antiglaucoma agents).

Systemic History

- History of arthritis or low backache (JRA, HLA – B27- related uveitis).
- History of fever or respiratory symptoms, gastro-intestinal symptoms, neurological symptoms, genital lesions.
- History of diabetes, hypertension and tuberculosis.
- History of exposure/IV drug abuse/blood trans-fusions.
- History of skin lesions (herpes zoster ophthalmicus, psoriasis).
- Details of prior systemic treatment.

Past Investigations

- Any recent investigations.
- Rheumatoid factor, antinuclear antibodies, ESR, Mantoux test, chest X-ray.
- If the above investigations have already been done in the past, the results can be recorded with the approximate date of the tests.

Medication

- Current medication (both topical and systemic).
- If the patient has discontinued the medications for the last few days it is useful to record when the patient last used the medication and what was the last dose at which the medication was stopped.

EXAMINATION

- Pinhole visual acuity.
- *Conjunctival congestion:* Type-circumciliary (need to differentiate between conjunctival congestion and circumciliary congestion).
- Any corneal opacity (if present corneal sensation should be tested for).
- Corneal edema.
- Keratic precipitates (fine/medium/large; distribution; fresh/old).
- Aqueous flare and cells (grading using SUN classification system as described below).
- Presence of posterior synechiae (preferable to draw the amount of pupillary dilation).
- Lens–cataractous or not.
- Intraocular pressure (if raised gonioscopy).
- Anterior vitreous cells (grading).
- Fundus examination (presence of cystoid macular edema and pars planitis, note disc cupping) .

Anterior Chamber

Flare (Protein in Aqueous)

- *Slit-lamp set to maximum intensity and magnification:*
  - Width of slit 1 mm
  - Length of slit 3 mm

Grading	Description
0	Complete absence
+	Faint - barely detectable
++	Moderate - iris and lens details clear
+++	Marked - iris and lens details hazy
++++	Intense - fixed coagulated aqueous with fibrin

Cells (Slit-Lamp Setting Same as for Flare)

- Inflammatory cells—small, spherical, glistening and nonpigmented (predominating lymphocytes and plasma cells) move with varying speed
- Macrophages—larger
- Pigment cells and granules—detected by their small size and color.

Grading (cells per field)	Grade
>1	0
1-5	0.5+
6-15	1+
16-25	2+
26-50	3+
>50	4+

INVESTIGATIONS

- First attack of nongranulomatous anterior uveitis in a patient with no systemic disorder—no investigations.
- Anterior uveitis secondary to herpes zoster ophthalmicus—no investigations.
- Traumatic anterior uveitis—no investigations.
- Recurrent attacks of nongranulomatous anterior uveitis—rheumatoid factor, antinuclear antibodies and ESR.

In addition to the above:

- If history is suggestive of recurrent uveitis with arthritis—*HLA B27.*
- If systemic steroids are being contemplated—chest X-ray.

- If history of exposure is present—VDRL, TPHA.
- If history of tuberculosis is present—Mantoux test.
- Granulomatous anterior uveitis—investigations to rule out sarcoidosis and tuberculosis:
  - Chest X-ray, Mantoux test, ESR, QuantiFERON TB GOLD test, SACE.

INITIAL TREATMENT

- Depending on the severity frequent doses of topical steroids (prednisolone acetate eyedrops as frequent as every 15 minutes)
- In the presence of glaucoma–to add antiglaucoma agents such as timolol 0.5 percent eyedrops if no contraindication is present
- Cycloplegics–strong cycloplegics are required in acute anterior uveitis
- If the pupil is mobile–homatropine eyedrops are required. If there are recent posterior synechiae–it is preferable to use atropine eyedrops to break the synechiae.
- In HLA-B27 related anterior uveitis–systemic steroids may be required, if unresponsive to topical steroids.
- Consultation and coordinated treatment with a rheumatologist, internist may be necessary in patients with systemic disorders.

FURTHER TREATMENT

Tapering of topical steroids over 4 to 6 weeks is done according to the response.

INTERMEDIATE UVEITIS

Intermediate uveitis was a term introduced by the International Uveitis Study Group (IUSG) as a part of an anatomic classification for uveitis. The intermediate zone of the eye is considered to be an area of the eye that includes the ciliary body, pars plana, choroid and peripheral retina as far posteriorly as the exit of the vortex veins. Intermediate uveitis is one in which inflammation involves this area of the eye. Pars planitis is described as the type of uveitis in which there is accumulation of inflammatory material in the region of the vitreous base and pars plana and is idiopathic.

CLINICAL FEATURES

Intermediate uveitis has no racial or genetic predisposition. It can occur at any age. It accounts for 10 to 39 percent of patients with uveitis. Patients complain of floaters, blurred vision or distortion of central vision.

SYMPTOMS

Usually unilateral or bilateral and wax and wane over many months. The external eye is often white and uninflamed.

SLIT-LAMP EXAMINATION

The anterior segment is quiet or has low-grade flare and cells with few keratic precipitates. Vitreous cells are always seen in the retrolental space. Fundus examination may reveal optic disc swelling, retinal edema, cystoid macular edema, prominent cellular infiltration and aggregation of inflammatory cells in the inferior vitreous cavity called as vitreous snow balls. Posterior vitreous detachment is common. In severe parsplanitis, significant vitreous traction may result because of inflammation induced fibrocellular proliferation. At times this can result in tractional and rhegmatogenous retinal detachment.

Characteristic Hallmark of Pars Planitis

* Presence of snow bank over the pars plana region, which is, white in color and may become vascularized. Usually snowbanks are confined to the inferior fundus. It may at times involve pars plana for 360°. These snowbanks may also be associated with neovascularization, tractional retinal detachment and retinoschisis. Chronic CME is the most common cause of visual loss and may at times become irreversible as a result of retinal pigment epithelial destruction. Macular hole formation can occur. There may be associated epiretinal membrane formation with macular edema. Patients may have secondary complications like cataract, glaucoma or vitreous hemorrhage.
* Intermediate uveitis may be associated with multiple sclerosis; it is diagnosed by taking a clinical history for symptoms of vertigo, ataxia, visual loss, paresthesia, weakness of sphincter dysfunction. It is necessary to recognize symptoms of demyelination and to refer to neurologists for further assessment.
* Sarcoidosis may be associated with intermediate uveitis and requires careful review of systems especially respiratory system to rule out the same.
* Vitreous cells with poor response to anti-inflammatory agents especially in the older age group may be a presentation of intraocular lymphoma.
* Ocular toxocarasis usually present as unilateral intermediate uveitis. Lyme's disease with features of erythema chronicum migrans, arthropathy may also present as intermediate uveitis.

INVESTIGATIONS

Investigation is guided by results of clinical assessment and review of systems. Angiography or optical coherence tomography (OCT) may be useful in patients with the vision of 6/12 or less to document macular edema and justify therapy.

The aim of each investigation is to rule in or rule out specific diagnosis.

MANAGEMENT

Management in intermediate uveitis is individualized and based on parameters like:
- Presence of unilateral or bilateral disease
- Visual acuity in each eye
- Severity of inflammation, presence of CME and threat to vision. Management decisions are clearly based on the level of visual acuity and presence of macular edema.

OPTIONS OF TREATMENT AVAILABLE

- Disease observation
- Medical therapy
- Surgical therapy

The four step therapy of Kaplan as a protocol consists of:
1. Local and systemic steroids.
2. Cryotherapy applied to snowbanks.
3. Pars plana vitrectomy.
4. Immunosuppression.

We use the following modified protocol of Kaplan:

Step 1: Local and Systemic Steroids

In patients with intermediate uveitis with complaints of severe floaters and vision of 6/12 or less, posterior subtenon injection of triamcinolone acetonide 40 mg/ml is used. If required this injection can be repeated after 4 to 6 weeks.

In patients who are unable to tolerate periocular steroids or those in which the disease does not responded to periocular steroids or those who have bilateral disease oral steroids prednisolone 1 mg/kg body weight is started along with oral calcium supplement and antacids.

Step 2: Immunosuppression
Final step involves use of immunosuppressives. Immunosuppressive drugs like cyclosporine, azathioprine and methotrexate or mycophenolate mofetil are recommended.

Azathioprine may be used in combination with steroids at the dose of 1–2 mg/kg body weight. Requires monitoring of bone marrow function and liver function test.

Cyclosporine A: 5 mg/kg in two divided doses daily is gradually tapered over by months to maintenance of 1–2 mg/kg. Low dose methotrexate at dosage of 7.5 to 15 mg per week is relatively safe and needs periodic monitoring of liver function and total white blood count and platelet count. Mycophenolate mofetil is given one gram twice daily.

Intermediate uveitis may become inactive and quiescent after a protracted course. Tight control of inflammation and close monitoring of the disease as well as its complications results in good visual recovery.

Step 3: Cryotherapy or Indirect Laser Photocoagulation
Failure of patient to respond to the above, cryotherapy is used, as described by Aaberg. It involves single freeze-thaw treatment of snowbanks. Cryotherapy may also be useful in patients with neovascularization in snowbanks. Indirect laser therapy can also be used in case of recalcitrant pars planitis.

Step 4: Pars Plana Vitrectomy
If cryotherapy fails or is by-passed, the third step involves pars plana vitrectomy to remove inflammatory debris in the hope that it will reduce visual loss resulting from macular edema.

POSTERIOR UVEITIS

A patient is labeled as posterior uveitis when the inflammation involves predominantly the posterior segment, i.e. retina, choroid or retina and choroid both.

History Taking in Posterior Uveitis

- *Common symptoms are:*
  - Blurring of vision
  - Marked loss of vision
  - Floaters
- *Relatively uncommon symptoms:*
  - Metamorphopsia
  - Micropsia
  - Macropsia
  - Scotoma
  - Ocular discomfort
  - Leukocoria (*Toxocara* in children).

Severe pain or photophobia as in anterior uveitis is not common. If a patient complains of severe pain around the eyeball please keep in mind posterior scleritis, which can often mimic posterior uveitis. A patient of posterior uveitis may not have any symptoms if the lesions are away from the macula.

- After taking the history of ocular disease, you should take history pertaining to cause of posterior uveitis. This can be done after fundus examination also
- Contact with pets (*Toxoplasma, Toxocara*)
- Oral and genital ulceration (Behcet's disease)
- Fever, weight loss, cough (Tuberculosis).

In case of suspicion of viral retinitis, one should rule out history of unprotected sex with commercial sex workers. This should be done mentioning that such personal history would help to make the diagnosis and treatment such history should be asked when patient is alone. Patient should be assured of the confidentiality. History of immunosuppression (drugs like corticosteroids, immunosuppressive drugs) and organ transplant is usually seen in cytomegalovirus retinitis.

Systemic History

Associated systemic diseases like diabetes, hypertension should be asked for:
- One should also note whether this is the first episode or is there a previous history.
- In case of previous history of posterior uveitis, the diagnosis, treatment given and its dosage, duration and the response is to be noted.
- In case patient had previous laboratory tests done, this should be noted in the file.
- Baseline visual acuity should be recorded with and without glasses.

OCULAR EXAMINATION

- This is done as usual in other case. Look for presence of anterior chamber reaction (aqueous cells in particular) carefully
- One should look for cells in anterior vitreous by slit-lamp examination. Presence of vitreous cells indicate inflammatory pathology and will rule out non inflammatory pathology like CSCR, metastatic tumor, ARMD.
- Once you have a fundus examination completed, first make a morphologic diagnosis, i.e. retinitis, choroiditis, chorioretinitis, retinochoroiditis.
- Certain posterior uveitis has characteristic features like toxoplasmic retinochoroiditis, which often seen around a previous scar, have head light in fog like appearance.
- Serpiginous choroiditis—which has got a geographic border.

- While the patient is on the slit-lamp, one can use +78 D or + 90 D lens to look at the lesions closely. Vitreous cells can also be identified by this examination.
- However it is best to have an indirect ophthalmoscopic examination. Here you should focus behind the lens to identify the vitreous haze, have an examination of whole retina.
- Find the lesions; first distinguish whether it is inflammatory or degenerative lesion.
- Lesion location, number (single, multiple) pattern, border should be noted. Particularly, if the lesion is close to the macula, whether fovea is involved or not should be mentioned.
- Always make a diagram.
- Identify the level of lesions choroidal, deep retinal, retinochoroidal.
- Active lesions will have ill-defined margin, yellow or cream colored.
- Healed lesions are well defined, pigmented.
- There are some lesions, which can be in between like resolving retino choroiditis.
- One should also look for involvement of optic nerve (papillitis).
- One should also look for associated retinal vasculitis.

INVESTIGATIONS

Once you make a clinical diagnosis, laboratory investigations are ordered to identify the etiology, confirm a clinical suspicion.

Common Laboratory Tests in Posterior Uveitis in Our Institute

- ELISA for *Toxoplasma,Toxocara*
- ELISA for HIV
- Mantoux test, chest X-ray, QuantiFERON TB Gold test (tuberculosis).

- Mantoux test, chest X-ray, serum angiotensin converting enzyme; lysozyme (sarcoidosis).
- VDRL and TPHA (syphilis).

Certain ancillary tests are done: Fundus photograph is always preferred to be taken in all cases of active posterior uveitis.

Indications:
- White dot syndromes
- Active or questionable active chorioretinitis
- Choroidal neovascular membrane
- Posterior scleritis
- There is no need to do FFA in healed choroiditis.

Indocyanine Green Angiography
Indications
- White dot syndromes
- VKH
- Sympathetic ophthalmia
- CNVM
- Questionable inflammatory choroidal lesions.

The immunosuppressive agents that we use commonly are azathioprine (50 mg 3 times/day) with low dose oral steroid (40 mg/day). While steroid can be tapered off, azathioprine can be continued for three to six months.

One may follow tablet azathioprine 50 mg 3 times/day for one to two months, 2 times/day for one to two months and 1 time/day for one to two months. One may choose other agents like methotrexate weekly, 15 mg on Sunday morning with folic acid tablet. Alkylating agents like cyclophosphamide 50 mg 2 times/day, i.e. 100 mg/day can be given. This can be gradually tapered off.

Cyclosporine is often preferred in Behcet's disease. The dosage is 5 mg/kg of body weight in two divided doses.

How soon to follow-up?

It is always better to see the response to treatment. So, follow up after one to two weeks to see response is needed. After that depending on the response, follow up after one to three months is needed.

Discussion with the patient

- Please explain the chance of recurrence.
- Active advice to report in case of development of scotoma or blurring of vision.
- In patient with choroiditis, it is always advisable to give home Amsler chart for noting down any change in the central field of vision.

Ultrasound

Should be done in suspected VKH, sympathetic ophthalmia and posterior scleritis.

MANAGEMENT

- In case of vision threatening inflammation, management can be started on the same day.
- One should rule out an infective etiology like *Toxoplasma* or tuberculosis.
- Noninfectious (immune mediated) uveitis are treated with systemic steroid and/or immunosuppressive agent.
- *Systemic steroid:* This is given at 1 mg/kg of body weight.
- One should rule out systemic infections like active TB, before putting on oral steroid by getting chest X-ray.
- *I/V methylprednisolone:* This is given in severe and vision threatening posterior uveitis. Dose in adults in 1 gm/day for three consecutive days (details enclosed).

Posterior sub-Tenon steroid: This is given if the lesion is causing macular edema or lesion is involving macula.

Immunosuppressive agent: This is given when there is no response to steroid by two weeks or patient has serious side effect (e.g. uncontrolled diabetes) due to steroid. In certain diseases like Behcet's disease and serpiginous choroiditis, immunosuppressive agents are always preferred.

PANUVEITIS

In panuveitis, both anterior and posterior part of the uveal tract is involved by the inflammation.

Common Panuveitic Condition

- Sympathetic ophthalmia
- Vogt-Koyanagi-Harada syndrome
- Sarcoidosis
- Behcet's disease
- Syphilis
- Idiopathic
- Lens induced uveitis.

HISTORY

Common Ocular Symptoms

- Marked dimness of vision
- Pain, redness and photophobia
- *History should be taken to identify any specific syndrome:*
  - Sympathetic ophthalmia (penetrating trauma, intraocular surgery)
  - Vogt-Koyanagi-Harada (VKH) disease (headache, meningism, hearing loss, alopecia, vitiligo, poliosis)
  - Sarcoidosis (erythema nodosum, lymphadeno-pathy, respiratory problem)
  - Behcet's disease (oral, genital ulcer).

OCULAR EXAMINATION

This is done as in any other case of uveitis.
Look for:
- KPs
- Aqueous flare, cells
- Iris nodules
- Synechiae
- Vitreous cells.

FUNDUS EXAMINATION

- Identify the vitreous inflammation (assess the degree).
- Optic nerve involvement (papillitis, papilledema).
- Secondary retinal detachment.
- Retinal, choroidal, retinochoroidal lesion.
- Dalen-Fuchs nodules (sympathetic ophthalmia).
- Retinal vasculitis (Behcet's disease sarcoidosis).
- Sunset glow fundus (Vogt-Koyanagi-Harada disease).

One should carefully examine pars plana to rule out severe pars planitis, which can mimic panuveitis.

Important Differential Diagnoses

- Endogenous endophthalmitis (history of intra-venous infusion, AIDS)
- Masquerade syndrome (elderly patient).

INVESTIGATIONS

- A patient of unequivocal case of sympathetic ophthalmia or VKH or Behcet's disease will not require any laboratory test.
- Other patients will require laboratory tests to rule out primarily tuberculosis, sarcoidosis, syphilis and HIV.
- Aqueous and vitreous tap should be done if suspicion of endogenous endophthalmitis or lens-induced uveitis exists.

Ancillary Tests

Ultrasound may be done in case of suspected VKH and sympathetic ophthalmia (diffuse choroidal thickening).

Fundus fluorescein angiography is often not required as the view is hazy, but can provide characteristic feature of early pinpoint hyperfluorescence and late confluent areas of staining in case of VKH.

MANAGEMENT

- Such patients require aggressive treatment. If infective etiology is ruled out, first-line of therapy is frequent topical steroid with mydriatic – cycloplegic agents (prednisolone acetate eyedrops every 1 hourly).
- Systemic steroid (oral prednisolone) usually given 1 mg/kg of body weight and tapered gradually according to response.
- Periocular depot steroid can be added.
- In case of Behcet's disease, immunosuppressive agents (cyclosporine, azathioprine) is preferred than oral steroid.
- In case of vision-threatening inflammation where infectious etiology is unlikely IV methylprednisolone 1 gm daily for three consecutive days can be given.
- Patient with VKH, sympathetic ophthalmia will require tapered dose of systemic steroid or immunosuppressive agents at least for nine months, sometimes a year or more.

PROGNOSIS

- Visual prognosis is good if treatment is started early and adequate dosage.
- Complication like cataract and glaucoma can occur.
- Periodic evaluation should be advised, as chance of recurrence is quite high.

SCLERITIS

SYMPTOMS

- Severe and boring eye pain.
- Usually gradual onset with red eye and insiduous decrease in vision.
- Recurrence is common.

CRITICAL SIGNS

- Inflammation of scleral, episcleral and conjunctival vessels.
- It can be sectoral or diffuse.
- Sclera may have a bluish hue (best seen in natural light).

OTHER SIGNS

Scleral nodules, peripheral keratitis, glaucoma, uveitis, exudative retinal detachment.

CLASSIFICATION

- *Anterior scleritis:*
  - Diffuse scleritis: Widespread inflammation of anterior segment
  - Nodular scleritis
- *Necrotizing scleritis with inflammation:*
  - Extreme pain
  - Sclera becomes transparent because of necrosis
- *Necrotizing scleritis without inflammation (Scleromalacia perforans):*
  - Almost complete lack of symptoms
  - Mainly seen in patients with long-standing rheumatoid arthritis
- *Posterior scleritis:*
  - Pain, tenderness, proptosis
  - Restricted extraocular movements
  - Can have exudative retinal detachment, disc swelling, retinal striae.

ETIOLOGY

- Fifty percent of the patients with scleritis have an associated systemic disease
- Common causes include rheumatoid arthritis, systemic lupus erythematosis, Wegener's granulomatosis, polyarteritis nodosa, tuberculosis, herpes zoster ophthalmicus.

WORK UP

- History
- Examination of sclera in all directions of gaze with adequate room light.
- Slit-lamp examination to look for any avascular areas of sclera.
- Dilated fundus examination.
- CBC, ESR, serum uric acid, RF, ANA, SACE level, VDRL, TPHA, ANCA testing especially c-ANCA for Wegener's granulomatosis, chest X-ray, Mantoux test, B-scan ultrasound to detect posterior scleritis.

TREATMENT

Treatment options include:
- Systemic nonsteroidal anti-inflammatory agents, e.g. indomethacin, diclofenac, ibuprofen. We usually give in active scleritis sustained release indomethacin tablet (75 mg) 1 tablet twice daily.
- Systemic steroids (1 mg per kilogram of body weight).
- Immunosuppressive therapy e.g. cyclophosphamide, methotrexate, azathioprine.
- Patients with necrotizing scleritis often need to be put on systemic steroids and immunosuppressive agents.
- In patients with infectious scleritis, treat with appropriate topical and systemic antibiotics.

FOLLOW-UP

Depends upon the severity of symptoms and the degree of inflammation. Decrease in pain is a sign of response to treatment even if inflammation appears unchanged.

RETINAL VASCULITIS

Retinal vasculitis is the term used to describe posterior uveitis of varying etiologies with involvement of retinal vasculature as a predominant presenting feature.

SYMPTOMS

- Asymptomatic
- Floaters
- Photopsia
- Metamorphopsia
- Diminution of vision.

SIGNS

- Active vascular disease is characterized by sheathing of the vessels. In sarcoidosis, characteristic "candle wax dripping" appearance is seen. Eales' disease characteristically involves the venules in the mid peripheral fundus.
- Vitreous cells
- Optic disc swelling
- Cystoid macular edema
- Associated cotton wool spots, retinal edema and hemorrhages
- Neovascularization of the disc or elsewhere.

CAUSES

- *Primary retinal vasculitis:* Eales' disease
- Retinal vasculitis associated with systemic inflammation, e.g. Behcet's disease, sarcoidosis, systemic lupus erythematosis, Wegener's granulomatosis.
- Retinal vasculitis associated with other ocular inflammatory conditions, e.g. pars planitis, acute retinal necrosis, cytomegalovirus retinitis.

- Retinal vasculitis associated with systemic or ocular infections, e.g. tuberculosis, syphilis, toxoplasmosis. Conditions like diabetic mellitus, severe hypertension and lymphomas can produce a picture that mimics vasculitis.

MANAGEMENT

- History
- *Slit-lamp examination:* Recurrent anterior uveitis with hypopyon is common in Behcet's disease.
- Fundus examination with indirect ophthalmoscopy and scleral depression. +78D/+90D examination to look for cystoid macular edema.
- *Fundus fluorescein angiography:* It may reveal active leakage from sheathed vessels with late staining of the vessel wall. It is particularly helpful in determining the flow pattern in inflamed vessels and detecting areas of capillary non-perfusion and neovascularization.
- *Other investigations include:* Total leukocyte count, differential leukocyte count, ESR, Chest X-ray, SACE levels, Mantoux test, serum lysozyme levels. Depending on the clinical picture, specific tests can be ordered like serum ANCA testing in cases of Wegener's granulomatosis.
  A young man presenting with repeated vitreous hemorrhages and periphlebitis should have Eales' work up as is done at our hospital.

TREATMENT

- For noninfectious causes of retinal vasculitis, systemic steroids are the mainstay of treatment. This is given at 1 mg/kg of body weight and is tapered 10 mg per week. Periocular steroids along with topical steroids may be required in certain cases.
- Immunosuppressive agents like cyclophosphamide or azathioprine may be needed in Wegener's

granulomatosis and in cases not responding to or requiring prolonged systemic steroids.
- Laser photocoagulation to manage neovascular complications.
- For infectious causes, specific treatment of underlying cause, e.g. tuberculosis, toxoplasmosis, acute retinal necrosis.

USE OF STEROIDS AND IMMUNOSUPPRESSIVE AGENTS

DOSAGE

The initial dose of steroids is 1 mg/kg body weight/day (usually 60-80 mg/day) orally. The dose has to be tapered over period of time with the tapering schedule being 60-80 mg/day for 1-2 weeks depending on severity of inflammation, followed by 50 mg/day for one week, then 40 mg/day for one week subsequently to decrease by 5-10 mg/week to reach 20 mg/day for one to two weeks following which the decrease is by 2.5-5 mg/week. It can be held at 10-15 mg/day for one month in case of indolent uveitis.

SIDE EFFECTS

Three major types of adverse effects are noted with therapeutic use of steroids.
1. Adrenal insufficiency following withdrawal of therapy due to continued inhibition of corticotropin releasing factor.
2. Hyperadrenocortisim–Cushing's syndrome
3. Activation of underlying disease process that has been suppressed prior to therapy.

Complications of Corticosteroid Therapy

Musculoskeletal	• Myopathy
	• Osteoporosis—vertebral compression fractures
	• Aseptic necrosis of the bone
Gastrointestinal	• Peptic ulceration (gastric)
	• Gastric hemorrhage
	• Intestinal perforation
	• Pancreatitis
Central nervous system	• *Psychiatric disorders:*
	– Insomnia
	– Nervousness
	– Mood changes

	• Maniac depressive psychosis
	• Schizophrenic psychosis
	• Suicidal attempts
	• Pseudotumor cerebri
Ophthalmic	• Glaucoma
	• Posterior subcapsular cataract
Cardiovascular and renal system	• Hypertension
	• Sodium and water retention-edema
	• Hypokalemic alkalosis
Metabolic	• Precipitation of clinical manifestations including ketoacidosis of genetic diabetes mellitus, hyperosmolar, nonketotic coma
	• Hyperlipidemia
	• Induction of centripetal obesity
Endocrine	• Growth failure
	• Secondary amenorrhea
	• Suppression of hypothalamic-pituitary-adrenal system
Inhibition of fibroplasia	• Impaired wound healing
	• Subcutaneous tissue atrophy
Suppression of immune response	• Superimposition of a variety of bacterial, fungal, viral and parasitic infection
Miscellaneous	• Increased urinary uric acid excretion
	• Increased serum protein binding of iodine
	• Hypocalcemic tetany—children
	• Spontaneous menstrual disorders

FETAL AND NEONATAL COMPLICATIONS (PREGNANCY)

Although pregnancy does not appear to increase the risk of adverse reaction to steroids, increased incidences of still births secondary to placental insufficiency have been noted.

Corticosteroids are excreted in breast milk and may cause inhibition of endogenous steroid production as well as growth suppression, therefore mothers receiving oral steroids should avoid breastfeed their infants. In case, steroid is absolutely indicated, we suggest the mother to feed the baby before intake of steroid and give a gap of three to four hours at least before the next breastfeed.

CHRONIC CORTICOSTEROID THERAPY

- Corresponding to the diurnal cycle, steroids are dispensed as a single dose in the morning after breakfast (before 9 AM).
- Replacement doses are given during acute stress situations such as trauma, infection, and surgery.
- Alternate day administration of steroids minimizes the typical cushingoid side effects associated with steroid therapy and in children, normal growth pattern can be maintained, which is not possible with daily steroid therapy. Alternate day therapy is usually given after initial treatment with everyday regime.

Most of the above mentioned side effects are reversible on stopping the steroid prescription.

INVESTIGATIONS DURING STEROID THERAPY

- Chest X-rays are done before starting steroid therapy to rule out pulmonary tuberculosis.
- Postprandial examination of blood sugar.

TERMINATION OF SYSTEMIC THERAPY

Tapering of steroid dosage is generally necessary for patients who have been on systemic therapy for more than seven to ten days. It is generally done by consolidation into a single dose/tapering and switching to alternate day therapy.

DRUG INTERACTIONS

Steroids inhibit the oxidation of opiates, barbiturates and thereby increase their effect.

Rifampicin, phenylbutazone, phenytoin may enhance the metabolism and decrease the effect of steroids. Response to anticoagulant therapy is reduced by concurrent administration of steroids.

DO'S AND DON'TS FOR THE PATIENT DURING STEROID THERAPY

- Do take antacid preparation one hour before food and before bed.
- Do ample exercise as it may help in overcoming the muscle wasting effects of the steroids.
- Do take a low sodium (salt) diet as it prevents hypertension associated with corticosteroid use.
- Do not overlook frequent mood changes or erratic behavior, it may be a side effect of the steroid, encourage family members to look for subtle behavioral changes and inform doctor if any.
- Do carry a medical identification card or wear a bracelet informing current medications. It may be useful in times of emergency such as accidents when adjunctive steroid supportive therapy might be required.
- Do inform your ophthalmologist about any other medication, which you are taking (for drug interactions).
- Do inform your physician about your recent prescription, in times of illness, it might be necessary to modify the steroid dosage.
- Do not become pregnant during the course of treatment.
- Do not hesitate to call on your doctor if you develop a side effect that you think might be related to the use of the steroid.

SITUATIONS IN WHICH STEROIDS SHOULD BE USED WITH CAUTION

- Diabetes mellitus
- Infectious disease
- Chronic renal failure
- Congestive heart failure
- Systemic hypertension.

SITUATIONS IN WHICH STEROIDS SHOULD NOT BE USED

- Peptic ulcer
- Osteoporosis
- Severe psychosis.

IMMUNOSUPPRESSIVE AGENTS IN UVEITIS

These drugs are used in severe ocular inflammation, which is sight threatening and which does not respond to conventional therapy. They play a role in modifying the response of the immune system of the body. These agents should be used in sufficient doses initially to control the inflammation and then tapered progressively after the inflammation subsides. Although these drugs are known to cause some serious side effects there might sometimes be no choice but to include these drugs in the treatment schedule. The drugs commonly used are:

Azathioprine (Azoran/Imuran): This drug is given orally in two or three divided doses per day. This to be used along with steroids. Side effects noted are:

- Bone marrow suppression
- Skin rash
- Arthralgia
- Fever
- Gastrointestinal symptoms.

One can get anemic and may be susceptible to infections. Hence blood counts are to be monitored every two weeks and patient should be closely followed up for any side effects of the treatment. The results of the blood counts are to be checked and if the total blood counts dropped below 3,000 or the platelet counts below 1,00,000, or if there is development of any infection in other parts of the body, the medicines have to be immediately stopped.

Cyclosporine (Sandimmune/Panimmune): This is a drug that is used for very severe inflammation threatening the vision. This medication is given in two-divided dose everyday. This drug may cause:

- Nephrotoxicity
- Hirsutism
- Gingivitis
- Dysesthesias
- Visual hallucinations
- Transient blindness
- Seizures.

Cyclosporine can alter the kidney functions. Hence kidney function tests like checking the blood urea, serum creatinine and blood pressure check has to be done every week. If abnormality in these tests are noted, the dose of the medication has to be reduced as required.

Cyclophosphamide (Cytoxan or Endoxan): This is a medication that is used in two divided doses per day in severe forms of uveitis. The usual dose is 50 mg twice daily. Side effects of this drug are:

- Bone marrow suppression
- Nausea
- Diarrhea
- Hemorrhagic cystitis
- Sterility
- Cardiac toxicity.

This medication can cause anemia and at times hematuria (i.e. blood in the urine). Patient is advised to drink 2 to 3 liters of water daily while on this drug.

Methotrexate (Neotrexate): The drug is given usually orally, but can be given subcutaneously. The drug can be given 7.5 to 15 mg per week. The drug to be taken once a day.

The side effect is hepatotoxicity (3%). It is effective in patients with sympathetic ophthalmia, cyclitis and severe juvenile rheumatoid arthritis related iridocyclitis. The routine tests done during follow up of patients on methotrexate are: chest X-ray, liver function test, blood count (total WBC and platelet).

Tablet folic acid (Folivit) 1 tablet daily to be given 3 days a week along with it.

Mycophenolate mofetil: 1000 mg twice a day, available as 250 mg and 500 mg capsules. Side effects include weight loss, gastrointestinal upset and bone marrow suppression. Mycophenolate mofetil has lesser side effects than other antimetabolites because they don't interfere with the salvage pathway of purine synthesis. Monitoring includes:

* Complete blood count - every month
* Liver function test (especially AST and ALT) every month.

Secondary malignancies have also been reported with this immunosuppressive medication.

However, please note that most of these complications listed above are rare and they need to be recognized and treated early. The above drugs should be prescribed after taking into account the benefits and risks of treatment. Patient should be advised to cooperate and take the medicines regularly for the control of the disease.

CATARACT SURGERY IN UVEITIS

Cataract is a common complication in patients with uveitis, especially those with chronic inflammation and long-term steroid therapy. The cataract surgery in uveitis is considered complicated because the surgical removal is more difficult than routine senile cataracts.

Surgical access is limited in these eyes due to posterior synechiae, pupillary sclerosis, pupillary membranes and excessive iris stromal or vascular fragility. They can have exuberant postoperative inflammatory response. The outcome of the surgery and the visual rehabilitation depends upon success of surgery itself, postoperative course and structural damage already caused by the pre-existing uveitis.

STRATEGIES FOR SUCCESSFUL MANAGEMENT OF CATARACT IN UVEITIS PATIENTS

Cataract surgery is generally deferred longer in uveitic eye than in normal eye.

Indications for Cataract Surgery

- A complicated cataract causing significant visual impairment.
- Cataract that impairs fundus examination in a patient with suspected fundus pathology.
- Cataract surgery in a patient with active uveitis is contraindicated except in the presence of phaco antigenic uveitis.

Preoperative Assessment and Patient Selection

- Visual potential may be restricted due to pre-existing complications of uveitis like cystoid macular edema, epiretinal membrane or glaucomatous optic atrophy.

- Visual potential can be assessed with potential acuity meter.
- Fundus fluorescein angiography and ultrasound can also provide useful information.
- Establishing an etiology and diagnosis of uveitis governs the surgical plan.
- Patients with Fuch's heterochromic iridocyclitis, intermediate uveitis and patients with uveitis, which has been quiescent for more than a year, are good candidates for intraocular lens implantation.
- Patients with juvenile rheumatoid arthritis or recurrent granulomatous anterior uveitis may be poor candidates for intraocular lens implantation.
- Patients with uveitis and secondary glaucoma do well with combined surgeries.
- In every case, good clinical judgment and patient selection is of utmost importance in the successful outcome of surgery.

Preoperative Management

- Tight control of inflammation for a minimum period of three months prior to surgery, which can be achieved with systemic, periocular, topical steroids or immunosuppressive if required.
- All inflammatory cells both in the anterior chamber and vitreous must be eliminated prior to surgery.
- Flare should not be used as guide post for inflammatory quiescence, as it cannot be eliminated. Flare simply denotes vascular incompetence of iris or ciliary body vessels as a result of recurrent inflammation.
- Good preoperative control of intraocular pressure.

Surgical Options

- Phacoemulsification with intraocular lens implantation or manual extracapsular cataract extraction with intraocular lens implantation is done in complicated cataracts with no posterior segment pathology.

- *Pars plana approach:* Lensectomy and vitrectomy is done in chronic uveitis of JRA. Intraocular lenses are relatively contraindicated.
- Combined phacoemulsification or extracapsular cataract extraction with vitrectomy done in patients with cataract with posterior segment pathology

Postoperative Management

- Frequent topical steroid are used and gradually tapered depending on postoperative inflammation.
- Systemic steroids are continued in gradually tapering doses over few weeks.
- Systemic immunosuppression may be rarely required, but may be used in severe postoperative inflammation.
- Cycloplegics are not required routinely, but are useful in eyes with fibrin reaction or with a tendency to synechiae formation.

Postoperative Complications

- Secondary glaucoma—intraocular pressure needs close monitoring and control.
- Cystoid macular edema—may be pre-existing or may occur following surgery.
- Posterior capsular opacification.
- Intraocular lens deposits.
- Reactivation of a pre-existing uveitis.

Conclusion

Successful rehabilitation of vision in uveitic cataracts is multifaceted challenge. Prudent case selection, absolute control of pre/postoperative inflammation, careful surgical planning, and meticulous surgery are essential for a good visual outcome.

INVESTIGATIONS IN UVEITIS

Why Laboratory Tests?

- To identify presumed autoimmune disease
- To identify specific uveitis entities
- To obtain diagnostic, prognostic and therapeutic directions.

STEPS BEFORE ORDERING INVESTIGATIONS

- Take uveitis oriented history
- Complete eye examination
- Identify anatomic location of the primary uveitis
- Get an overall systemic evaluation
- Compare clinical characteristic with known uveitis entities
- Shortlist etiological possibilities
- First-order first relevant lab investigations
- Then order extensive investigations if the eye condition is refractory to treatment.

When you do not Need to Order for any Lab Tests

- Fuch's heterochromic iridocyclitis
- Traumatic uveitis
- First attack of acute anterior uveitis
- Sympathetic ophthalmia
- Vogt-Koyanagi-Harada's disease.

What Lab Tests you should do Always?

- ESR
- Total and differential white blood cell count.

Raised ESR

- *Noninfectious causes:*
  - Collagen disorder
  - Sarcoidosis

- *Infectious cases:*
  - Tuberculosis
  - Syphilis
  - Toxocara.

SEROLOGICAL TESTS

- Antinuclear antibody (ANA)
- Rheumatoid factor (sclerouveitis only)
- Anti-neutrophilic cytoplasmic antibody (Wegener's granulomatosis).

Rheumatoid Factor

- Positive in RA, scleritis, sclerouveitis
- Negative in JRA, ankylosing spondylitis.

Antinuclear Antibodies Positive

- Ankylosing spondylitis
- JRA
- SLE
- Dermatomyositis
- Scleroderma
- Sjögren's syndrome.

Serological Tests for Syphilis

- VDRL – state of activity.
- *FTA-ABS:* High degree of sensitivity and specificity.
- Order both in suspected syphilis.

ELISA Test from Serum

- *Toxoplasma*
- *Toxocara*
- HIV.

ELISA for TB from Serum

- Very little diagnostic value due to high prevalence of systemic TB.

ELISA for Toxoplasmosis

- Sensitivity 100 percent
- Specificity 50 percent
- Always correlate clinically.

When should you Order ELISA for HIV

- Herpes zoster ophthalmicus in a young person
- Herpes zoster ophthalmicus involving more than one dermatome in any age group
- Endogenous endophthalmitis
- Multiple cotton wool spots.

Human Leukocyte Antigen

- Present on 6th chromosome
- Class I, II and III—A, B, C and D.

HLA Typing is not Required Routinely

- HLA A29—Birdshot retinochoroidopathy
- HLA B5 (51)—Behcet's disease
- HLA B27—nongranulomatous recurrent anterior uveitis.

HLA—B27 Positive Anterior Uveitis

- Acute onset
- Unilateral, recurrent
- Fibrin, hypopyon
- More complications like synechiae, CME
- Needs aggressive treatment
- Educate about symptoms
- Follow-up at close intervals.

Investigations for Sarcoidosis

- Serum angiotensin converting enzyme (SACE)
- Serum lysozyme
- Serum calcium, inorganic phosphorous.

SACE

- Normal level 8 to 52 units.
- Patients on systemic steroid may have false negative value

- All cases of granulomatous uveitis
- Intermediate uveitis
- Choroid nodules.

Skin Tests

- Mantoux test—tuberculosis
- Kveim test for sarcoidosis (is no longer done).

Ancillary Investigations

- *X-ray chest:*
  - Tuberculosis
  - Sarcoidosis
  - All patients prior to oral steroid therapy
- X-ray lumbosacral region
- CT scan
- MRI
- Gallium scan
- *Angiography:*
  - Fundus fluorescein angiography (FFA)
  - Indocyanine green angiography (ICG).

Role of FFA

- For diagnosis.
- To determine extent of involvement.
- To follow disease process.
- To identify the complications in multifocal choroiditis, GHPC, postinflammatory SRNVM, CME in pars planitis.

Ancillary Tests in Uveitis

- *Ultrasound:*
  - B scan
  - Ultrasound biomicroscopy

Findings

- Choroidal thickening (VKH, sympathetic ophthalmia)
- Posterior scleritis
- Vitreous opacities

- Cyclitic membrane
- RD, choroidal detachment.

Pathologic Study

- Anterior chamber paracentesis
- Vitreous biopsy
- FNAB
- Chorioretinal biopsy.

Indications for Pathologic Study

- Lens induced uveitis
- Infectious etiology
- Parasitic infestation
- Endophthalmitis
- Masquerade syndrome.

Nongranulomatous Anterior Uveitis

- Blood test TLC, DLC, ESR.
- Serological test-ANA.
- HLA B27.
- Chest X-ray.
- X-ray sacroiliac joint.

Granulomatous Anterior Uveitis

- Blood test TLC, DLC, ESR
- Mantoux test
- VDRL
- FTA-ABS
- Serum ACE
- Serum calcium
- Serum lysozyme
- QuantiFERON TB Gold test.

Investigations of Uveitis in Children below 15 Years

- ESR
- ANA
- Mantoux test
- X-ray chest

- VDRL
- X-ray knee joint.

Investigations in Adults

- ESR
- HLA B27
- Mantoux test
- X-ray chest
- VDRL
- Sacroiliac joint.

Speciality Consultations to be Sought

- Internal medicine
- Pediatrics
- Rheumatology
- Neurology
- Chest physician
- Dermatology.

INVESTIGATIONS FOR TUBERCULOSIS

INDICATIONS

- Granulomatous uveitis
- Subretinal abscess
- Choroidal tubercles
- Clinical evidence of pulmonary/systemic tuberculosis.

BASELINE

- Chest X-ray
- Mantoux test
- QuantiFERON TB Gold test.

SECOND LEVEL INVESTIGATIONS

- Chest physicians opinion
- *Biopsies:* Ocular/Nonocular sites.

Chest X-ray

Chest X-ray is ordered for tuberculosis as well as sarcoidosis in uveitis. Chest X-ray film suggestive of tuberculosis should show calcified tuberculomas, multinodular infiltrates with cavitation in the upper segment of either lungs or a miliary pattern. However, tuberculosis may produce any form of pulmonary radiographic abnormality especially in immunocompromised patients.

The diagnosis of ocular tuberculosis is to be considered in all patients of chronic iridocyclitis, chronic granulomatous iridocylitis.

Mantoux Test

Mantoux test is done by intradermal injection of 0.1 ml of PPD antigen into the volar surface of the forearm. The report in analyzed after 48 hours. The important feature is the presence of induration, not erythema. Induration of 10 mm in diameter or greater is considered positive. Five to nine millimeter is doubtful and less than 5 mm is negative. The Mantoux test is not advisable as a routine screening test among patients with uveitis. About 60 to 70 percent of normal healthy Indian peoples have positive Mantoux test. The Mantoux test should be done in patient with symptoms or signs suggestive of tubercular uveitis/granulomatous uveitis or patient having pulmonary tuberculosis with symptoms such as cough, fever or cachexia, past history of weight loss, night sweat, history of chronic or recurrent pulmonary infection or past exposure to the tuberculosis, or if the chest X-ray made the diagnosis more likely.

Though 67 percent of tubercular uveitis shows a positive response to the Mantoux test, 33 percent of tubercular uveitis can have a negative Mantoux test. Therefore, clinical judgement needs to be used while making the diagnosis of tuberculosis.

QuantiFERON TB GOLD Test

The QuantiFERON TB Gold test is approved for use in the United States (Food and Drug Administration, 2007) and in many countries around the world. It is an objective, single visit blood test that measures the IFN-gamma response of T cells to *Mycobacterium tuberculosis* antigen. The QuantiFERON test has not been found superior to tuberculin skin test in sensitivity for use as a screening test or first-line study in TB- related uveitis, bit it is more specific than tuberculin skin test. It is less affected by BCG vaccination.

Other Investigations

- AC tap for
    - Direct smear (Ziehl-Neelsen stain or fluorescent acid fast stain)
    - Culture
    - Polymerase chain reaction

- Sputum test
- Urine culture
- Lymph node biopsy
- Concentrating the mycobacteria using centrifugation or other technique could be expected to increase the yield of positive results.
- Fluid specimens (such as aqueous or vitreous) should be immediately inoculated into a liquid medium or aqueous (Lowenstein Jensen media) for primary isolation of mycobacteria. Culture should be kept for a minimum of eight weeks and examined weekly for evidence of growth.

Molecular Biologic Techniques

In recent years, the polymerase chain reaction has been developed to identify the mycobacteria. These methods include uses of a heat stable enzyme, DNA polymerase to amplify mycobacterial DNA from clinical samples. Several studies have demonstrated the utility of PCR for *Mycobacterium tuberculosis* in clinical samples including samples of aqueous humor and vitreous from patients with suspected intraocular tuberculosis. PCR is more rapid and sensitive than culture and conventional Ziehl-Neelsen technique. We have investigated the use of PCR for detection of *Mycobacterium tuberculosis* in case of suspected cases of intraocular tuberculosis. Both IS6110 and nested PCR are done for this purpose.

INTERPRETATION OF LABORATORY TESTS FOR TOXOPLASMOSIS

- Ocular toxoplasmosis can frequently be diagnosed clinically on the basis of its characteristic chorioretinal scar and inflammation.
- Serologic testing confirms the clinical diagnosis of toxoplasmosis.
- Following laboratory tests can be employed.

ELISA Test for Antibodies to *Toxoplasma Gondii* from Serum (Serological Test)

As is true for several laboratory tests, a negative result for antibodies to toxoplasmosis is sometimes more informative than a positive result. All patients with ocular toxoplasmosis should have some evidence for an immune response to toxoplasma. Thus the absence of antibodies to toxoplasmosis may exclude the diagnosis of toxoplasmosis. There are three caveats to this dictum:

- An absent antibody response could represent a laboratory error
- An immunocompromised patient could have a minimal immune response
- Because the infection may be confined to the eye, the systemic expression of the immune response could be meager.

A primary infection with toxoplasmosis is suggested by:

- Flu like symptoms
- A positive IgM antibody titer to toxoplasma
- A fall in IgM or a marked decrease of IgG titer several months after the onset of ocular inflammation.

Anterior Chamber Paracentesis for Toxoplasmosis

The supernatant fluid after spinning down of cellular components within the aqueous humor should be subjected to ELISA for the detection of specific antibodies. Tests to determine the level of specific immunoglobulins (IgE) may also be of help. The local production of specific antibodies within the ocular fluids is an important indication for the possible etiology. The decision regarding ELISA titers obtained from the aqueous humor is evaluated against the titer of similar antibodies detected in the serum. There exists a passive transfer of antibodies into the ocular fluids from the serum. Therefore, the Goldmann – Whitmer (Whitmer – Desmonts) coefficient must be calculated.

- A coefficient higher than three can be considered as a positive indication for the active production of specific antibodies within the eye.

Polymerase Chain Reaction for Toxoplasmosis

Definitive diagnosis rests on pathologic demonstration of cysts or free organisms. It requires polymerase chain reaction (PCR) amplification or rRNA gene of *T. gondii* from aqueous samples. This test when used in concurrence with ELISA test can increase the sensitivity of diagnosis of *Toxoplasma gondii* infection.

INTERPRETATION OF LABORATORY TESTS FOR HUMAN IMMUNODEFICIENCY VIRUS

- Testing for human immunodeficiency virus (HIV) infection is done in cases when HIV infection is suspected clinically such as in CMV retinitis, young patients with squamous cell carcinomas, endogenous endophthalmitis, and herpes zoster ophthalmicus
- The primary means of documenting HIV infection is by HIV antibody testing and viral culture. Viral cultures are both expensive and time consuming, so antibody testing is the method of choice for rapid and inexpensive confirmation of HIV exposure
- In our institute, the Tri-Dot™ and Immunocomb™ tests are used for detection of HIV antibody. These are rapid HIV antibody assays
- Rapid tests are increasingly in use as they can be performed easily as special equipments are not needed and generally require 30 to 90 minutes. Most rapid tests are the variations of enzyme immunoassays (EIA) with various combinations of HIV 1 and HIV 2 antigens
- Apart from the false-negative results during the "window" period, false-positive reactions may occur in conditions such as autoimmune diseases, renal failure, cystic fibrosis, multiple pregnancies and vaccinations for hepatitis B
- A reactive serum should be tested again in duplicate and if reactive is considered as confirmed
- However, antibody testing alone is not diagnostic for AIDS
- Western blot or indirect immunofluorescence tests on the reactive serum are the further confirmatory tests if required. The western blot technique is one that uses electrophoresis to separate viral antigens and measures serum antibody reaction to specific viral proteins (core and envelope proteins).

INTERPRETATION OF LABORATORY TESTS FOR CYTOMEGALOVIRUS

- Testing for cytomegalovirus (CMV) is ordered in certain conditions such as viral retinitis (acute retinal necrosis, CMV retinitis)
- The diagnosis in these conditions is primarily clinical and the serology is of supportive value alone
- The ELISA test is done in our institute to detect antibodies to CMV
- Raised IgM titers are suggestive of recent infection
- Raised IgG titers are only suggestive of past exposure to the virus
- CMV is a ubiquitous organism and many normal individuals have serum antibodies to CMV; hence the interpretation of the tests has to be done in correlation with the clinical findings
- Aqueous and vitreous aspirate is of more diagnostic value. Anterior chamber tap should be done in case there are cells in anterior chamber. Material should be submitted for immunofluorescence study for all three herpes virus (HSV, HZV and CMV). Immunofluorescence report is ready on the same day within few hours. In addition, material should be submitted for PCR for all three herpes viruses (HSV, HZV and CMV). PCR report is ready after 24 hours. Both immunofluorescence and PCR are highly sensitive and specific tests.

ANTERIOR CHAMBER TAP

- Inform the patient regarding the procedure.
- Clean the eye and periorbital region with povidone iodine eye solution.
- Put a drop of antibiotic eyedrops and then a drop of anesthetic (lidocaine or paracaine) eyedrops.
- Take a sterile cotton bud, put few drops of paracaine solution over it and place the bud over the site of paracentesis.
- Put the lid speculum.
- Under good illumination, using 26G to 30G needles, the anterior chamber is entered through clear cornea avoiding damage to iris and the lens.
- About 0.3 to 0.4 cc of aqueous is collected.
- The aqueous can be studied microbiologically (direct smear, immunofluorescence, culture), cytopathology (lens induced uveitis), molecular biologic study (polymerase chain reaction). Angiotensin converting enzyme can also be assessed in aqueous.

PERIOCULAR STEROID INJECTION IN UVEITIS

INDICATIONS

- Severe anterior uveitis not responding to topical steroids
- Intermediate uveitis
- Any uveitis associated with cystoid macular edema
- Unilateral posterior uveitis
- Severe uveitis not responding to topical and systemic steroids
- Prior to surgery in a uveitic eye to prevent peri-operative/postoperative inflammation, e.g. cataract surgery
- Uveitic patients in whom compliance to topical treatment is doubtful
- Patients in whom complications have developed due to systemic steroids or complications due to oral steroid are to be avoided.

CONTRAINDICATIONS

- Scleritis
- Ocular toxoplasmosis.

SITE OF INJECTION

- Subconjunctival
- Anterior sub-Tenon
- Posterior sub-Tenon
- Retrobulbar.

Due to the complications associated with other methods only posterior sub-Tenon is routinely given.

PREPARATIONS

Highly water soluble and short acting (6-12 hours)
- Dexamethasone sodium phosphate
- Hydrocortisone sodium succinate.

Moderately water soluble and intermediate acting (2-3 days)
- Triamcinolone diacetate
- Methylprednisolone.

Poorly water soluble and long acting (3 weeks – 3 months)
- Triamcinolone acetonide (Tricort or Kenacort)
- Triamcinolone hexacetomide.

The side effects due to these agents are related not only to the drug itself but also due to the preservative used, e.g. retinal toxicity, lenticular toxicity is more common when some agents are used. Considering these issues triamcinolone acetonide have been found to be the safest agents among these agents.

POSTERIOR SUBTENON INJECTION IN UVEITIS

Procedure

- Superotemporal is the most commonly chosen quadrant
- Liberal topical anesthesia applied–four percent lignocaine or proparacaine eyedrops
- Upper eyelid is elevated and cotton swab soaked in topical anesthetic drops placed over injection site for about 15 to 20 seconds
- One milliliter of triamcinolone acetonide is taken in a 2.5 ml disposable syringe attached with 26 gauge 5/8 inch needle
- Bulbar side and not forniceal side of the conjunctiva is chosen because of more visibility and more firm attachment to Tenons capsule in this area; the subtenons space can be easily reached
- Initially lid is pulled and the needle is introduced with the bevel towards the globe
- The needle is kept as close to the globe as possible.
- Broad side-to-side movements are made that are parallel to the circumference of the globe and the needle is moved posteriorly so that in case sclera gets engaged it can be easily recognized, as the globe also will start making similar movements

- Once the needle is fully introduced plunger is withdrawn to see if the needle is in any vessel
- 0.5 to 0.75 ml is slowly injected
- No white swelling should be visible if the drug has been given in the posterior sub-Tenon space.

Complications

- Increase in IOP and glaucoma
- Globe perforation and attendant complications like:
  - Hypotony
  - Vitreous hemorrhage
  - Retinal detachment
  - Choroidal hemorrhage
  - Endophthalmitis
  - Phthisis.
- Accidental intravascular injection can lead to embolism to retinal and choroidal circulation
- Skin depigmentation
- Fat atrophy
- Repeated injections can cause extraocular muscle fibrosis and proptosis
- Ptosis.

SUBCONJUNCTIVAL INJECTION OF MYDRICAINE

INDICATION

To break fresh posterior synechiae.

DRUGS

- Phenylephrine hydrochloride (Drosyn) 10%
- Homatropine hydrobromide (Homide) 2%
- Adrenaline
- Lignocaine (Xylocaine) 2%.

PREPARATION OF 0.4 ml OF MYDRICAINE

- Phenylephrine hydrochloride   - 0.1 ml
  (Drosyn) 0.5%
- Homatropine hydrobromide   - 0.2 ml
  (Homide) 0.2%
- Adrenaline   - 0.1 ml

0.1 ml of 0.4 ml mydricaine thus prepared is given sub-conjunctivally close to the site of synechiae.

PREPARATION OF 0.5% DROSYN

- 0.1 ml of 10% Drosyn + 0.9 ml of 2% Xylocaine = 1% Drosyn
- 0.5 ml of 1% Drosyn + 0.5 ml of 2% Xylocaine = 0.5% Drosyn.

PREPARATION OF 0.2% HOMIDE

0.1 ml of 2% Homide + 0.9 ml of 2% Xylocaine = 0.2% Homatropine.

COMPLICATION

Subconjunctival hemorrhage.

INTRAVENOUS ACYCLOVIR
(ACIVIR OR ZOVIRAX)

METHOD OF PREPARATION

- 1500 mg/m^2/day for 14 days (7–21) days in three divided doses
- Each 10 ml vial contains 500 mg of acyclovir
- Contents to be dissolved in 10 ml of sterile water or bacteriostatic water containing benzyl alcohol yielding a final concentration of 50 mg/ml (pH-11).

DOSAGE

- 5 mg/kg over one hour
- 15 mg/kg/day
- Should be added to appropriate intravenous solution (DNS/RL) for one-hour infusion
- Average 70 kg adult - 60 ml of fluid/dose (50 mg/ml preferable)
- Shelf life of diluted fluid 12 hours
- Refrigeration might cause precipitation, which re-dissolve in room temparature
- *Monitor:* Kidney function test.

INTRAVITREAL GANCICLOVIR INJECTION IN CMV RETINITIS

PREPARATION

To prepare 400 mg of ganciclovir:
- Vial of ganciclovir contains 500 mg of the drug
- Add 10 ml of sterile water for injection to 1 vial
  1 ml = 50 mg
  0.8 ml = 40 mg
- Add 0.2 ml of sterile water for injection
  0.1 ml = 4 mg = 4000 µg
- Add 0.9 ml of sterile water for injection
  0.1 ml now contains 400 µg of ganciclovir.

PRECAUTIONS

The drug can cause local irritation. Avoid inhalation or direct contact of the powder or reconstituted solution with the skin or mucous membranes. In case of accidental contact with the skin or mucous membrane wash thoroughly with soap and water. For eye exposure, rinse thoroughly with plain water.

DOSAGE

400 to 1600 µg.

COMPLICATIONS

Iatrogenic retinal break
Lens touch
Vitreous hemorrhage
Retinal detachment
Endophthalmitis
Suprachoroidal detachment.

STEPS OF INJECTION

- Clean the eyelids and the periorbital area with cetrimide solution.

- Apply topical proparacaine/xylocaine eye drops.
- Insert wire speculum.
- Place a cotton bud tipped and soaked with topical proparacaine/xylocaine over the site of injection
- Measure the distance from the limbus with calipers:
  - Phakic eyes   - 3.5 mm from the limbus
  - Pseudophakic eyes   - 3.0 mm from the limbus
  - Aphakic eyes   - 3.0 mm from the limbus or at the limbus
  - Children   - 2.5 to 3.0 mm from the limbus (procedure under general anesthesia)
- The intravitreal injection is prepared as directed
- The injection is given with 30 gauge needle directed towards the mid vitreous cavity
- After withdrawing the needle completely a tipped cotton bud is applied to the site of the injection
- In case of raised IOP following the injection, an anterior chamber paracentesis should be done
- Topical ciprofloxacin is applied
- Wire speculum is removed and the eye is patched for two hours.

6

Neuro-ophthalmology

- Neuro-ophthalmological Evaluation
- Evaluation of a Swollen Optic Disc
- Optic Neuritis
- Anterior Ischemic Optic Neuropathy
- Papilledema
- Diplopia
- Anisocoria
- III Nerve Palsy
- IV Nerve Palsy
- VI Nerve Palsy
- Myasthenia Gravis
- Functional Visual Loss/Malingering
- Orbital Cellulitis
- Traumatic Optic Neuropathy
- Toxic Amblyopia
- CT and MRI in Ophthalmology

NEURO–OPHTHALMOLOGICAL EVALUATION

HISTORY

- Visual loss—onset/progression/severity/with or without pain
- Double vision—type/constant/horizontal or vertical, oblique
- *Headache:*
  - Severity/laterality/incidence
  - Associated features—nausea/vomiting/giddiness/aura/field defects
- *Field defects involving:*
  - Central/peripheral/superior/inferior
  - Floaters
- Involuntary movements of eyeball—onset/oscillopsia
- Blackouts—frequency/duration/complete/partial
- Color vision defect—congenital/acquired
- Drooping of lid (Ptosis)—unilateral/bilateral/onset/progression/associated features-variability/diplopia/jaw winking/glare.
- Protrusion of eyeball (Proptosis)—onset/progression/associated features—redness/variability with posture/pain/vision loss/diplopia/sensation loss/headache.
- Miscellaneous—speech and hearing defect/numbness/weakness of limbs/tremors/facial weakness/gait imbalance.

PAST HISTORY

Trauma/diabetes/hypertension/ATT and chronic drugs use/alcoholism/smoker/IHD/thyroid disease/myasthenia/cerebral palsy/radiotherapy/chemotherapy.

EXAMINATION

- Best corrected visual acuity
- Pupils—size/reaction to light and near/RAPD-trace to 4+
- Color vision by Ishihara plates
- Confrontation visual field—type of field defect
- Ocular movements—primary position/movement restriction/severity/gaze palsy
- Lid position—ptosis/retraction
- Proptosis evaluation—type—axial or eccentric/ retrobulbar resistance/pulsatile/amount/measure with Hertel's exophthalmometer/bruit.
- Nystagmus—manifest or latent/jerky or pendular/ horizontal, vertical or tortional/amplitude/ direction/nullpoint/dampening on convergence/ nystagmoid movements.
- Cranial nerves examination
- CNS examination—cerebellar signs/higher functions/extrapyramidal signs/motor and sensory examination
- Anterior segment examination—conjunctival corkscrew vessels in proptosis, anterior uveitis, postsurgery signs.
- *Fundus examination:*
  - Media and vessels
  - Disc—blurring of margins/edema/pallor/ hyperemia/blood vessel changes
  - Retinopathy—diabetic/hypertension

EVALUATION OF A SWOLLEN OPTIC DISC

Step 1: Is this true disc edema or pseudopapilledema?
Step 2: If this is true disc edema, then is it papilledema (due to raised intracranial pressure).

Pseudopapilledema vs true disc edema

Pseudopapilledema	True disc edema
1. Hyperopia	1. No significant refractive error
2. Small discs	2. Normal disc size
3. Cup absent	3. Cup present until late stage
4. Peripapillary retinal edema absent	4. Peripapillary retinal edema – Paton's lines present
5. Anomalous vessels – Multiple branchings on/close to disc – Anomalous loops pointing to disc	5. No anomalous vessels – Tortuous vessels – Peripapillary hemorrhage/ exudates
6. Vessels clearly visible on disc surface	6. Vessels partly obscured by overlying nerve fiber edema
7. Lumpy or irregular disc surface	7. Uniformly elevated disc

When in doubt...

- *Check BP:* Systemic/malignant hypertension is a cause of bilateral disc edema. Patients may be asymptomatic.
- *Ultrasound:* To rule out optic nerve head drusen: High spikes at optic nerve head even at low or zero gain settings.
- *FFA:* Autofluorescence at optic nerve head due to drusen. No disc leak in pseudopapilledema.

If true disc edema...is there optic nerve function impairment?

- Usually impaired optic nerve function: optic neuropathies
    - Optic neuritis (uni- or bilateral involvement)
    - AION (uni- or bilateral involvement)
    - Compressive (usually unilateral only)

- *Usually normal optic nerve function:*
  - Papilledema (almost always bilateral involvement)
  - Passive disc edema due to local causes, e.g. disc edema in central retinal vein occulsion (CRVO).

OPTIC NEURITIS

HISTORY

Ocular (Unilateral or Bilateral)

- Sudden visual impairment over several hours to 1 to 2 days (rarely a week). Extent of impairment may vary from very mild to NPL
- Pain or discomfort on ocular movements, especially on up gaze
- Color desaturation
- Central scotoma.

Systemic

- URI
- Prodromal viral fever
- Focal neurological deficits
- Sever physical exertion or excessive heat exposure.

PAST HISTORY

- Similar visual impairment improving well either spontaneously or with steroid treatment
- Focal neurological deficits
- Vaccination in children.

EXAMINATION FINDINGS

Ocular

- *Visual acuity (VA):* Impairment (rarely VA may be 6/6 or NPL)
- *Color vision:* Impaired
- *Ocular motility:* Pain or discomfort on ocular movements (especially up gaze)
- *Pupil:* Relative afferent pupillary defect (RAPD) always present in unilateral or asymmetric bilateral involvement
- *Fundus:* Normal or edematous optic nerve head
- *Confrontation fields:* Central scotoma/altitudinal/generalized sensitivity reduction.

Systemic

CNS: Focal motor, sensory or cerebellar deficits. Other cranial nerve palsies.

INVESTIGATIONS
Ocular

- Humphrey visual fields 30-2 threshold OU
- *Other tests of optic nerve function:* Contrast sensitivity, VEP. These are useful in cases of mild or doubtful optic neuritis mostly RBN to aid in diagnosis.

Systemic—Depends on Clinical Findings

- First episode of a unilateral isolated idiopathic optic neuritis in a patient aged 20 to 40 years:
  - No investigations
- *Bilateral optic neuritis:*
  - Complete hemogram
  - ANA
  - VDRL
  - X-ray PNS (if sinusitis is suspected)
  - Aquaporin-4 antibody–NMO specific antibody – aid in differentiating MS/NMO
- *Suspicion of multiple sclerosis:*
  - Clinical situations—recurrent optic neuritis, sequential optic neuritis, or optic neuritis with associated focal neurological deficits.
  - Magnetic resonance imaging (MRI) (brain and optic nerves) with contrast to look for MS plaques.
  - CSF analysis especially to look for oligoclonal bands.

TREATMENT
Treatment is Case Specific
IV Methylprednisolone

- *Indications:*
  - All optic neuritis with significant visual loss $\leq$ 6/12

- – Recurrent optic neuritis
- – Optic neuritis with hyperintense signals on MRI.
- Referral to neurologist for evaluation (MRI with gadolinium, CSF) and treatment.
- *Steroid clearance:*
  - – History of TB, diabetes mellitus, hypertension, malignancy or
  - – Check chest X-ray, postprandial blood sugar (PPBS), BP
  - – Also include ECG and serum electrolytes.
- *Treatment is inpatient with cardiac monitoring:*
  - – Intravenous methylprednisolone (IVMP) 1 gm/day in divided doses for 3 days
  - – This may or may not be followed by a course of systemic steroids with a regimen as mentioned above.

No Treatment

Indication:
- First episode of unilateral, isolated idiopathic optic neuritis with mild visual impairment (VA $\geq$ 6/12)
- Neurological evaluation.

FOLLOW-UP

- After a 2 to 3 days and then 1 week of treatment
- Typical optic neuritis should show some signs of improvement within a week of treatment
- Continue treatment regimen with longer follow-up periods. Repeat visual fields after completion of treatment.

ATYPICAL OPTIC NEUROPATHY (NOT DEMYELINATING)

Features

- Bilateral rather than unilateral
- Gradual onset rather than sudden
- Slowly progressive rather than improvement, i.e. response to steroids is nil or poor
- Recurrence while tapering steroids (steroid dependent optic neuropathy)

- Other ocular (e.g. intraocular inflammation) or neurological signs.

Management

- Complete neurological evaluation—refer the patient to a neurologist.
- Neuroimaging (always, preferably MRI with contrast).
- CSF analysis (if necessary).

NEURORETINITIS

- Neuroretinitis is an inflammation of the optic disc with adjacent retinal inflammation. Some cases of neuroretinitis are associated with a particular infectious disease, whereas others occur as an apparently isolated phenomenon, designated as 'Leber's idiopathic stellate neuroretinitis'. Neuroretinitis is a type of optic neuritis that is not associated with multiple sclerosis.
- Clinical features—acute, unilateral, painless loss of vision. The degree of color deficit is usually more than the visual loss. Presence of relative afferent papillary defect and a centro-coecal scotoma points towards optic nerve inflammation. A macular star figure composed of hard exudates appears within days to weeks and becomes even more prominent as the disc swelling resolves. Inflammation of the anterior and posterior segment of the eye may be associated.
- Fundus fluorescein angiography—demonstrates a diffuse disc swelling and leakage of dye from vessels on the surface of the disc. The macular vasculature is essentially normal.
- The infectious diseases, which cause neuroretinitis include cat-scratch disease, Lyme disease, leptospirosis and secondary and tertiary syphilis. If it develops as a part of the syndrome of syphilitic meningitis, the neuroretinitis is usually bilateral and associated with evidence of meningeal irritation and

multiple cranial neuropathies. Neuroretinitis is also commonly (50%) associated with an antecedent viral infection. Proposed causative agents include herpes simplex, hepatitis B virus, and herpes viruses associated with acute retinal necrosis. *Toxoplasma*, *Toxocara* and *Histoplasma* are also suggested to be causative agents.

- Appropriate serologic testing, of all granulomatous and infective etiology and analysis of cerebrospinal fluid and neuroimaging are desirable in patients with a history of systemic infection.

- Treatment depends on the underlying etiology. It is a self-limited disorder with a good prognosis. Over 8 to 10 weeks the optic disc swelling resolves. The macular exudate progresses over about 8 to 10 days, remains stable for several weeks before gradual resolution starts which occurs over 6 to 12 months. Most patients in due course recover good visual acuity.

BIBLIOGRAPHY

1. Ormerod LD, Dailey JP. Ocular manifestations of cat-scratch disease. Curr Opin Ophthalmol. 1999;10(3):209-16. Review.
2. Casson RJ, O'Day J, Crompton JL. Leber's idiopathic stellate neuroretinitis: differential diagnosis and approach to management. Aust NZJ Ophthalmol. 1999; 65-9. Review.
3. Reed JB, Scales DK, Wong MT, Lattuada CP Jr, Dolan MJ, Schwab IR. *Bartonella henselae* neuroretinitis in cat scratch disease. Diagnosis, management, and sequelae. Ophthalmology. 1998;105(3):459-66.
4. Parmley VC, Schiffman JS, Maitland CG, Miller NR, Dreyer RF, Hoyt WF. Does neuroretinitis rule out multiple sclerosis? Arch Neurol. 1987;44(10):1045-8.
5. Dreyer RF, Hopen G, Gass JD, Smith JL. Leber's idiopathic stellate neuroretinitis. Arch Ophthalmol. 1984;102(8):1140-5.

ANTERIOR ISCHEMIC OPTIC NEUROPATHY

Differentiate Between Arteritic and nonarteritic Type

- Arteritic anterior ischemic optic Neuropathy (AION): Emergency
- Nonarteritic AION is not an emergency.

ARTERITIC AION

- Ocular emergency
- Age 50+
- Associated with temporal arteritis.

Symptoms

Ocular

- Sudden profound visual loss (sometimes no perception of light, NPL)
- Unilateral but may become bilateral in hours to days.

Systemic

- Headache
- Jaw claudication
- Proximal muscle and joint pain
- Anorexia
- Fever
- Weight loss
- TIAs and/or stroke.

Signs

- *Visual acuity:* Profound visual loss, NPL not uncommon
- *Color vision:* Profoundly impaired
- *Ocular motility:* Usually normal; occasionally VI nerve palsy
- *Pupil:* Gross RAPD
- *Anterior segment:* Normal; signs of ocular ischemia

- *Fundus:* Pale optic disc edema, infarcted disc, cilioretinal artery occlusion occasionally
- *Confrontation:* Altitudinal field defect or fields generalized loss.

Systemic

- Painful, pulseless thickening of superficial temporal artery
- Carotid pulsations may be reduced in certain cases.

Investigations

Systemic

- Westergren ESR—very high, often over 100 mm/1 hour. {Normals: Males: $0.5 \times$ age; females: $0.5 \times$ (Age + 10)}, TLC, DLC
- C reactive protein elevated
- Vasculitis work-up
- *FFA:* Delayed choroidal filling, patchy perfusion defects
- Duplex scan of carotid arteries
- Temporal artery biopsy in selected situations.

Ocular

Especially important for fellow eye:
- Humphrey 30-2 threshold test OU especially important for fellow eye.
- Color vision.

Treatment

- Emergency
- *Aim:* To save the fellow eye.

IV Methylprednisolone

- Urgent steroid clearance—history of TB, diabetes mellitus, active infection of any kind.
- Check CXR, PPBS, BP. Include ECG and serum electrolytes.
- Treatment is inpatient with cardiac monitoring.
- Intravenous methylprednisolone (IVMP) 1 gm/day in divided doses for 3 days.

- This may or may not be followed by a course of systemic steroids—Tab Prednisolone 1 to 1.5 mg/kg/day as a single dose after breakfast with antacid cover.
- Rheumatology referral.

FOLLOW-UP

- Oral steroids have to be continued until symptoms abate and ESR returns to normal levels.
- Gradual taper of steroids with frequent periodic monitoring of ESR.
- Treatment may continue for 3 to 6 months or sometimes even 1 year.

NONARTERITIC AION

- Age 40 to 60
- Associated with systemic hypertension, diabetes mellitus, hypercholesterolemia.

Symptoms

- Sudden painless visual impairment, usually unilateral
- No associated systemic or prodromal symptoms.

History

- Systemic hypertension
- Diabetes mellitus
- Hypercholesterolemia
- Can follow cataract surgery occasionally.

Signs

- *Visual acuity:* Moderate-to-profound visual loss. NPL rare
- *Color vision:* Moderately impaired
- *Ocular motility:* Normal
- *Pupil:* Gross RAPD
- *Anterior segment:* Normal
- *Fundus:*
  - Characteristic altitudinal pallor/hyperemia/pale disc edema/hyperemic disc edema

- Fellow eye: Small crowded disc with absent cup– "disc at risk".
- *Confrontation:* Altitudinal field defect fields (usually inferior) or generalized loss.

Investigations
Ocular

- Humphrey 30-2 threshold test OU
- Color vision.

Systemic

- PPBS
- Blood pressure
- Lipid profile
- Rheumatoid arthritis (RA)/antinuclear antibody (ANA)/Antiphospholipid antibody/homocysteine.

Treatment

- Conservative management
- In cases of profound visual impairment and acute disc swelling, a short course of systemic steroids may be tried with guarded visual prognosis, if there are no absolute contraindications to steroid therapy.

Follow-up

Check the following:
- VA
- Fundus examination of discs
- Visual fields.

NATURAL COURSE

- VA may remain stable or improve by 1-2 Snellen lines.
- *Watch for worsening:* Progressive AION
- Warrants further investigation—complete hemogram, vasculitis work-up, neuroimaging to rule out a compressive lesion
- A possible indication for optic nerve sheath decompression (ONSD).

PAPILLEDEMA

Bilateral optic nerve head edema *due to raised intracranial pressure.*

HISTORY
Ocular

- Asymptomatic
- Impairment of optic nerve function (in late stage papilledema) characterized by:
  - Amaurosis fugax for a few seconds only
  - VA loss which can deteriorate rapidly over a few weeks.
- Binocular diplopia.

Systemic

- Asymptomatic
- Symptoms of raised intracranial pressure— headache, vomiting
- Symptoms of focal neurological deficits (e.g. VII and VIII nerve involvement in acoustic neuroma).

EXAMINATION FINDINGS
Ocular

- *Visual acuity:* Usually normal except in late stages
- *Color vision:* Usually normal except in late stages
- *Ocular motility:* Usually normal or VI nerve palsy (binocular diplopia or esodeviation especially for distance)
- *Pupil:* Normal, unless there is asymmetric impairment of optic nerve function
- *Fundus:*
  - Bilateral optic disc edema.
  - Secondary optic atrophy in late stages
- *Confrontation fields:* Normal, enlarged blind spot in early stages or generalized impairment/constricted fields in later stages.

Systemic

Central nervous system: Focal motor, sensory or cerebellar deficits or other cranial nerve palsies.

INVESTIGATIONS

- Fundus photographs of discs with 2x magnification—useful for documentation and follow-up.
- Visual fields—Humphrey 30-2 OU.
- *CT or MRI brain:*
  - To check for any intracranial mass lesion
  - Attenuated ventricles in benign intracranial hypertension.
- *CSF analysis:*
  - Record opening pressure
  - Other routine CSF study.
- Other tests—directed at detecting causes of benign intracranial hypertension—decision individualized.

TREATMENT

- *Referral to neurosurgeon* (in case of brain tumor) or *neurophysician* (in case of benign intracranial hypertension)
- Consider *optic nerve sheath decompression* if medical treatment of benign intracranial hypertension is ineffective and optic nerve function is progressively deteriorating.

FOLLOW-UP

- VA
- Fundus examination of discs
- Visual fields–Humphrey visual fields 30-2 OU.

DIPLOPIA

Double vision is a frequent symptom seen in neuro-ophthalmic disease. Sometimes patients complain of blurry vision instead of true diplopia.

ASK

- Whether double vision is *monocular or binocular*
- *Monocular diplopia*—causes are cataract, astigmatism, corneal scars, keratoconus, tear film irregularities, subuxated lens, iris atrophy, large or sector iridectomy, vitreous or retinal disease and in hysteria or malingering.
- If binocular—ask whether the diplopia is horizontal, vertical or torsional.
- Ask the patient in which direction of gaze is the diplopia worse—right, left, up, down, right and up, right and down, left and up, left and down, or distance or near.
- Ask for diurnal variability and fatigability of diplopia suggestive of myasthenia.
- Detailed history about mode of onset, duration of onset, associated pain, history of strabismus in childhood, history of trauma, neurological symptoms such as dysphagia or weakness, underlying systemic illnesses such as hypertension, diabetes, cerebrovascular disease, cardiac atherosclerotic disease, and multiple sclerosis. History of smoking or alcohol intake should also be elicited.

EXAMINATION

- Look for obvious misalignment, ptosis, head turn or face turn, proptosis, nystagmus and eyelid swelling.
- Check the best corrected visual acuity. Duochrome and worth four-dot test should be done. Check for

diplopia with Snellen's chart also. Binocular diplopia may also result from anisometropia.

- Examine the extraocular movements—ductions, versions and vergences. Saccades (horizontal and vertical) and smooth pursuit movements should also be checked.
- Cover/uncover, alternate cover, Hirschberg, Krimsky's, prism bar cover test and Maddox rod should be done in all cardinal positions of gaze. Incomitant deviations are suggestive of a neurological problem. Comitant deviations are suggestive of a longstanding childhood problem. Forced duction test should be done in case restrictive pathology is suspected.
- Pupil examination is a must
- Diplopia and Hess charting should be done to document the deviation and the underlying muscular dysfunction.
- Check for convergence insufficiency inpatients with asthenopic problems.
- Examine all other cranial nerves.

MANAGEMENT

- If the cause is neurological then the extraocular muscle, which is involved, should be documented. It requires neuroimaging preferably MRI scan to look for any intra cranial cause.
- For restrictive diplopia due to orbital causes such as thyroid ophthalmopathy, order an ultrasound of the orbits to look for extra ocular muscle thickening, retro bulbar mass lesion, etc. One may also order for CT scan of the orbit to document the same.
- Cases suspected to have myasthenia are referred to the neurologist for investigation and management.
- Ischemic ocular motor palsy due to diabetes/ hypertension usually resolves spontaneously within 3 to 6 months. Such patients may be

temporally asked to patch one eye. Inpatients with minimal deviation prisms may be tried. If diplopia/squint is not improving beyond this period then one may consider neuroimaging.

- Ocular misalignment which remains stable for 6 months may be considered for squint correction
- In children ocular motor palsies have a potential for developing strabismic or visual deprivation amblyopia, which should be treated by alternate daily patching between the eyes.
- If underlying intracranial cause such as tumor or aneurysm is established the case should be referred to the neurosurgeon, neurologist or neuroradiologist, as appropriate.

Horizontal Diplopia (Major Causes)

- 6th nerve palsy
- 3rd nerve palsy
- Convergence insufficiency
- Internuclear ophthalmoplegia
- Myasthenia gravis.

Vertical Diplopia (Major Causes)

- 4th nerve palsy
- 3rd nerve palsy
- Thyroid ophthalmopathy
- Myasthenia gravis
- Skew deviation.

ANISOCORIA

Evaluate the size, shape, and reaction to light and near of both pupils with the indirect ophthalmoscope.

Check if the anisocoria is more in the light or dark.

If more in the light:
- Look for limitation of adduction, elevation, depression, or ptosis—III nerve palsy
- *Check the slit lamp for:*
  - Sphincter tears—traumatic mydriasis
  - Vermiform segmental contraction of the pupillary sphincter—Adie's pupil.

Pharmacological testing in case of doubt/to confirm diagnosis:
- Pilocarpine test
- Instill diluted pilocarpine eyedrops (0.125%) in both eyes:
  - Pupil constricts—Adie's pupil
  - Does not constrict—advanced Adie's/III nerve palsy/pharmacological dilation.

    Perform test with normal strength pilocarpine in both eyes:
    - ◆ Pupil constricts—III nerve palsy
    - ◆ Pupil does not constrict—pharmacological dilatation.

If more in dark:
- Use 1:1000 adrenaline and look for dilation
  - If yes—Horner's syndrome
  - If no—pharmacological constriction.

MANAGEMENT
- Adie's pupil—evaluate knee jerk reflexes—dark glasses/bifocals if needed
- 3rd nerve palsy—MRI with MRA scan to look for compressive lesion
- Pharmacological—call patient for review after two weeks to recheck pupils
- Traumatic mydriasis—provide dark glasses/bifocals
- Horner's syndrome—chest X-ray, CT scan neck/head.

III NERVE PALSY

SYMPTOMS

- Drooping of the upper lid
- Binocular diplopia.

SIGNS

- Ptosis
- Eye turned "down and out"
- Restricted elevation, adduction and depression
- Nuclear III—check for bilateral ptosis or contralateral superior rectus impairment.

HISTORY

Diabetes mellitus, systemic hypertension, vasculitis.

CHECK FOR

Ocular

- Pupil sparing or involvement—any anisocoria worse in bright illumination?
- IV and VI nerve function
- Variability (myasthenia)
- Possibility of restrictive palsy (thyroid ophthalmopathy)—FDT.

Systemic

- Contralateral hemiparesis
- Contralateral hemitremor
- *Other neurological signs:* Headache, vomiting, etc.

INVESTIGATIONS

Hess and diplopia charting.

MANAGEMENT

Pupil Spared

- Evaluate diabetes mellitus (DM) and hypertension (HT)

- Conservative management
- Occlusion.

Pupil involved

- MRI with MRA
- Neurological opinion
- Occlusion (temporary), prisms or surgery (depending on degree of deviation once it is stabilized for 6 months).

Manage as Pupil Involved

- Multiple cranial nerve involvement
- Aberrant regeneration
- Pseudo-pupil sparing—concomitant sympathetic involvement.

IV NERVE PALSY

SYMPTOMS
- Binocular vertical diplopia
- Head tilt.

SIGNS
- Head tilt to opposite side of palsy
- Chin down
- Eye hypertropic
- Evaluation of vertical diplopia with three-step-test
- In IV nerve palsy
- Hypertropia will be worse on contralateral horizontal gaze and ipsilateral head tilt
- Any other neurological signs–check.

HISTORY
- Duration of head tilt—check old photos
- Diurnal variation—myasthenia
- FDT—restrictive palsy (orbital trauma, thyroid ophthalmopathy)
- Head trauma
- DM, HT.

INVESTIGATIONS
- Hess and diplopia charting
- If congenital IV nerve palsy is suspected—check old photos and test for vertical fusional amplitude, which will be quite large (about 8–10 PD).

MANAGEMENT
- If vasculopathic (DM/HT)—conservative management (temporary occlusion)
- *Trauma:* Prisms or surgery depending on degree of deviation once it is stabilized.
- Nonresolving IV nerve palsy which is not congenital or post-traumatic–MRI ± MRA.

VI NERVE PALSY

SYMPTOM

Horizontal binocular diplopia.

SIGN

Impairment of abduction.

Check for other cranial nerve/neurological involvement:

- *VI, papilledema:* Raised intracranial pressure (Tumor or PTC)
- *III, IV, V, VI, sympathetic:* Orbit or cavernous sinus lesion
- *V, VI:* Middle cranial fossa lesion
- *VI, VII, VIII:* CP angle lesion
- *VI, VII, VIII, sympathetic:* Dorsal pontine lesion
- *VI, VII, VIII, sympathetic, contralateral hemiparesis:* Ventral pontine lesion.

Isolated VI nerve palsy is nonlocalizing:
Consider MRI if not improving within 3 months and myasthenia and restrictive palsy have been excluded.

INVESTIGATIONS

- Hess and diplopia charting
- DM, HT
- MRI—for nonresolving palsy, or other neurological signs.

MANAGEMENT

- Treat the cause
- *Diplopia:* Patching (temporary), prisms or surgery (depending on degree of deviation).

MULTIPLE CRANIAL NERVE PALSY

Involvement of more than one of the following nerves: II, III, IV, V, VI.

LOCATION OF LESION

- Orbit
- Cavernous sinus

Check for diabetes mellitus (mucormycosis), immunocompromise.

INVESTIGATIONS

Orbital, PNS and neuroimaging—CT or MRI.

MANAGEMENT

Treat the cause.

MYASTHENIA GRAVIS

Most common causes of acquired unilateral and bilateral ptosis:
- Myasthenia gravis is a disease characterized by muscle weakness and fatigability attributable to decreased ACh receptors at neuromuscular junctions.
- Incidence is more in young females and older male patients.
- All ocular symptoms and signs are highly variable in nature and usually do not follow any classical pattern. Usually improve with rest and worsen on exertion, especially towards evening.
- There is no set pattern of extraocular muscle involvement it can be from isolated muscle to total ophthalmoplegia mimicking INO/gaze palsies/ nerve palsies.

CLINICAL SIGNS
- *Fatigue test:* Prolonged up gaze results in gradual lowering of eyelids.
- *Enhancement of ptosis:* Worsening of ptosis on one side when opposite eyelid is elevated. This seesaw mechanism is related to Hering's law of equal innervation.
- *Cogan's lid twitch sign:* When patient is instructed to look down for 10 to 20 seconds and then make a vertical saccade back to primary position, the upper lid elevates and droops slowly or twitches several times before settling.
- *Ice test:* Useful in patients with ptosis ice cubes to be kept over the lids for 2 minutes and then ptosis assessed-improvement in ptosis (>2 mm) is suggestive of myasthenia gravis (by measuring PF).
- Orbicularis oculi weakness observed during gentle eyelid closure as abnormal. Widening of palpebral fissure, initially patient is able to achieve eyelid apposition but later due to rapid fatigue patient appears to peek at the examiner-peek sign.

- Generalized features are weak expressions, dysarthria, and nasal regurgitation of liquids.

MANAGEMENT

The role of the ophthalmologist is indeed clinical diagnosis and management of ocular complaints related to myasthenia gravis. The patient is referred to the neurologist for treatment of the condition. Treatment by the ophthalmologists:

- Lid crutches for ptosis and patching for diplopia are good conservative measures.
- Chronic myasthenia with stable deviation and stable diplopia may be referred to the squint clinic for considering surgical correction of squint.

Investigations by Neurologist

- *Tensilon test (Edrophonium chloride)*
- *Repetitive nerve stimulation studies:* Shows decremental response in myasthenia gravis.
- *Single fiber electromyogram:* Suggestive of increase jitter and is highly sensitive for myasthenia gravis.
- *Antiacetylcholine receptor antibody assay:* RIA using human ACh receptor to detect antireceptor antibodies is a standard diagnostic test for myasthenia gravis.

Treatment by Neurologist

- *Cholinesterase inhibitors:* Pyridostigmine (Mestinon) –widely used–onset of action is within ½ hour and peaks at 1 to 2 hours. Starting dose 30 mg every 4 hours even can increase up to 120 to 150 mg every 4 hours.
- Oral corticosteroids are most effective for ocular myasthenia.
- Azathioprine and cyclosporine are other alternative modes of immunosuppression.
- Lid crutches for ptosis and patching for diplopia are good conservative measures.
- Chronic myasthenia with stable deviation and stable diplopia may be referred to the squint clinic for considering surgical correction of squint.

FUNCTIONAL VISUAL LOSS/ MALINGERING

- Denotes symptomatic and measured loss of vision that is unassociated with an identifiable lesion of visual pathway.
- Malingering implies willful alteration of subjective symptoms to secure secondary gain, e.g. adolescents before exams, workers after injury at work.
- *Types of patients:*
  - Deliberate malingerer
  - Worried impostor
  - Impressionable exaggerator
  - Suggestible innocent
- Diagnosis is suggested when examiner can demonstrate that patients behavior and responses to testing are inconsistent with an organic lesion.
- The technique to identify functional visual loss (FVL) patients depends on the level of visual loss they claim.

CLINICAL EXAMINATION

- *Observation:* Truly blind persons always proceed cautiously and avoid the furniture, etc. but FVL individuals knowingly bump into objects.
- *Proprioception tests:* Truly blind patients can do these without difficulty as these do not require vision but FVL patients will often not be able to do them, e.g. ask the patient to sign his name.
- *Mirror test:* When a large mirror is rocked in front of a normal person an involuntary nystagmoid movement results because of forced fixation on the mirror image. A patient with FVL will be unable to avoid this movement provided the patient is looking at the mirror.
- *Surprise test:* Suddenly if examiner makes a face or makes shocking actions, etc. and observes the

patient's response, a change in the patient's look is suggestive of malingering. Used in severe bilateral FVL.

- *Pupils:* Totally blind eye has nonreactive pupil to light, only cortical blindness is associated with intact pupillary reactions. So if a patient claims of total blindness with intact pupillary response and no evidence of cortical blindness, suspect malingering. In case of unilateral vision loss, a relative afferent pupillary defect (RAPD) is usually present.
- *Duochrome test:* The letters correspond to visual acuity of 6/12 and better. Used to test uniocular FVL.
- *Wort four-dot test (WFDT):* Appreciation of four dots indicates reasonably good vision in both eyes.
- *Prism shift test:* A normal prism shift occurs in presence of binocular vision. The prism is placed in front of alleged bad eye, if there is good vision in that eye a compensatory movement of both eyes towards apex of prism followed by convergence movement of fellow eye back to center occurs.
- *Fogging:* This technique involves blurring the good eye with lenses while patient views Snellen's chart binocularly. The acuity achieved represents the function of supposed bad eye. Higher plus lenses (+10D) are better than other lenses.
- *Visual fields:* Commonly seen field defects in FVL patients are:
  - Constricted fields
  - Tubular fields
  - Spiraling
- *Pattern visual evoked potential:* Provides valuable information about acuity level. But FVL patients can voluntarily alter the amplitude and latency of P100 peak by defocusing or looking away from the stimulus.

TREATMENT

This is mostly based on the physician's encouragement to patient reassuring that there is no major problem. Placebo treatment like prescribing low power glasses, various drops, contact lenses, etc. may improve vision in FVL patients.

ORBITAL CELLULITIS

IT IS AN OPHTHALMIC EMERGENCY

Infection of the soft tissues posterior to the orbital septum. In children it is usually associated with an upper respiratory infection.

Sources of infection include contiguous spread from sinuses (the most common source), face, lid, and oropharynx, from foreign bodies such as an orbital implant or from trauma, secondary to septicemia, from infected intraorbital structures like dacryocystitis, dacryoadenitis and panophthalmitis.

CAUSES

- Bacterial, fungal, parasitic infections
- *H. influenzae* is the common pathogen encountered in children. In debilitated adults, fungal infections such as mucormycosis may be seen.

CLINICAL FEATURES

Acute orbital cellulitis presents with:

Ocular

- Abrupt onset of pain
- Eyelid edema
- Conjunctival hyperemia
- Chemosis
- Proptosis (axial or non-axial)
- Diplopia
- Ptosis
- Ophthalmoplegia
- Severe visual loss (orbital apex lesions)
- Choroiditis
- Optic neuritis.

Systemic

Fever, malaise, leukocytosis, sinusitis.

CLASSIFICATION

Orbital cellulitis is classified into five groups namely:
1. Group 1—Preseptal cellulitis
2. Group 2—Orbital cellulitis
3. Group 3—Subperiosteal abscess
4. Group 4—Orbital abscess
5. Group 5—Cavernous sinus thrombosis.

COMPLICATIONS

Exposure and neurotropic keratitis, conjunctival prolapse, secondary glaucoma, septic uveitis and retinitis, exudative retinal detachment, optic neuropathy and panophthalmitis.

INVESTIGATIONS

- Basic hemogram, blood sugar, urine routine, pus culture/sensitivity.
- X-ray of paranasal sinuses—shows mucosal thickening, sinus opacification, and air fluid levels.
- Ultrasonography (B-scan) is sensitive in identifying lesions in the anterior or medial orbit.
- CT scan—more clearly demonstrates the precise location, extent of inflammatory process and source of infection such as sinusitis or foreign body.

MANAGEMENT

- The main aim of treatment is to prevent the development of meningitis and cavernous sinus thrombosis.
- Patient should be immediately handled on emergency basis at any hour of the day without delay. The following should be checked—visual acuity, pupils, extraocular movements, degree of proptosis and fundus and cranial nerve examination.
- Accurate grouping of the disease should be done in the first 24 to 48 hours. One should look for a systemic focus of infection.

- Patient should be immediately hospitalized. In case patient is debilitated with multiple systemic problems case to be immediately referred to an appropriate center for management.
- Urgent ultrasonography of the eye and orbit and CT scan of the brain, orbit and paranasal sinuses should be done. In case systemic infection is suspected blood culture should be ordered.
- Appropriate high dose intravenous antibiotics should be started. Cefuroxime is the first choice antibiotic (100 mg/kg body weight per day in 3 to 4 divided doses).
- Start Inj. Claforan 1 gm twice daily together with Inj. gentamycin 80 mg twice daily and Inj. metrogyl 100 ml twice daily.
- Alternatives include cloxacillin (100 mg/kg body weight in four divided doses) and chloramphenicol (75 mg/kg body weight per day in 4 divided doses).
- For fungal infections intravenous amphotericin B can be used. Antibiotics should be continued till signs of orbital inflammation subside.
- For prevention of complications—corneal protection with lubricants, antibiotics for the conjunctiva, temporary frost suture.
- Surgical drainage should be done in cases of demonstrable abscess or sinus infection (to coordinate with an ENT surgeon) that is compromising ocular function. In cases that present with panophthalmitis consider evisceration of the eye after a second opinion.
- Nasal decongestants, painkillers may be added.
- Careful and complete periodic follow-up is a must to ensure adequate recovery. This includes visual acuity, neurological assessment, extraocular movements, pupils, fundus and degree of proptosis. CT scan or ultrasound may be repeated to ensure resolution of infection.

TRAUMATIC OPTIC NEUROPATHY

It is optic neuropathy that is temporally related to blunt or penetrating head trauma that results following road traffic accidents, fall from a height or from frontal impact by falling debris, assault, stab wounds and gunshot wounds. May result following iatrogenic injury such as endoscopic sinus surgery or orbital surgery. Rarely results from orbital hemorrhage (retrobulbar hemorrhage) or orbital emphysema.

They are divided into:
- Direct injury that results from orbital or cerebral trauma that transgresses normal tissue planes to disrupt the anatomic and functional integrity of the optic nerve, e.g. bullet penetrating orbit. Vision loss is severe, immediate and recovery is unlikely.
- Indirect injury usually results from blunt trauma to the forehead that results in transmission of force through the cranium to the restrained intra-canalicular portion of optic nerve. Vision loss may be delayed and recovery is poor.

They are classified into 3 types:
- Optic nerve avulsion—ophthalmoscopic appearance consists of a partial ring of hemorrhage or the avulsion can be seen as a dark crescentic area.
- Anterior optic neuropathy—injury within 10 mm of the globe. Central retinal artery occlusion or vein occlusion may occur.
- Posterior optic neuropathy—injury posterior to entrance of central retinal artery or vein.

CLINICAL FEATURES
- Vision varies from no perception of light to 6/6. Associated field defect is present—altitudinal, central, paracentral, centrocecal. Injury to intracranial optic nerve produces hemianopic field

defect. Relative afferent pupillary defect is present in unilateral injury. Multisystem trauma or serious brain damage with loss of consciousness may be present.

- In some cases no evidence of orbital or ocular trauma is seen. Others may have periorbital or ocular hemorrhage, ecchymosis or laceration.

Investigations

- Visual evoked potential—helps in assessing optic nerve function in an unresponsive patient.
- CT scan orbit and brain—look for optic canal fracture fragments which can be impinging on the nerve.
- MRI—helps in evaluating intracranial abnormalities, can detect subtle hemorrhage of the optic nerve or its sheath.

Management

- Respiratory and cardiovascular resuscitation and stabilization are the first priority. Care of the patient may need a team approach. Treatment is based on the United States National Acute Spinal Cord Injury Study. Within 8 hours of injury patients should receive intravenous methylprednisolone at the rate of 30 mg/kg loading dose followed by a continuous infusion of 5.4 mg/kg/hour for 48 hours.
- If vision does not improve in 48 hours, optic nerve decompression may be considered. Cases with bony fragments impinging on the optic nerve will need decompression and evacuation of optic nerve sheath hematoma.
- Some cases can improve on their own without treatment.

BIBLIOGRAPHY

1. Van Stavern GP, Biousse V, Lynn MJ, Simon DJ, Newman NJ. Neuro-ophthalmic manifestations of head trauma. J Neuroophthalmol. 2001; 21(2):112-7.

2. Kountakis SE, Maillard AA, El-Harazi SM, Longhini L, Urso RG. Endoscopic optic nerve decompression for traumatic blindness. Otolaryngol Head Neck Surg. 2000;123(1 Pt 1):34-7.

3. Pomeranz HD, Rizzo JF, Lessell S. Treatment of traumatic optic neuropathy. Int Ophthalmol Clin. 1999; 39(1):185-94. Review.

4. Steinsapir KD. Traumatic optic neuropathy. Curr Opin Ophthalmol. 1999;10(5):340-2. Review.

5. Foster BS, March GA, Lucarelli MJ, Samiy N, Lessell S. Optic nerve avulsion. Arch Ophthalmol. 1997; 115(5):623-30.

6. Steinsapir KD, Goldberg RA. Traumatic optic neuropathy. Surv Ophthalmol. 1994;38(6):487-518. Review.

TOXIC AMBLYOPIA

- The term 'toxic amblyopia' and the related term 'tobacco-alcohol amblyopia' refer to one of the most frequently considered toxic or nutritional deficiencies that lead to optic neuropathy. A number of toxins injure the optic nerve and lead to a bilateral, slowly progressive visual loss.
- Tobacco-alcohol amblyopia results from the relative role of cyanide {from tobacco} and low levels of vitamin B_{12} brought about by poor nutrition and poor absorption associated with alcohol consumption. Deficiencies of B_{12}, other B vitamins and, in particular, folic acid are known to result in a similar clinical picture.
- Toxins established most clearly as producers of an optic neuropathy include carbon monoxide, clioquinol, cyanide, ethambutol, hexachlorophane, isoniazid, lead, methanol, plasmocid. Certain factors, e.g. impaired renal function in patients on ethambutol may increase the risk and severity of toxic optic neuropathy.
- The agents which are less evidently toxic to the optic nerve are carbon disulfide, chloramphenicol, pheniprazine, quinine, and thallium.
- Toxic injury to the papillomacular bundle is fundamental to the problem.
- Patients initially complain of an inability to read, see traffic signs, or appreciate face details of acquaintances. The visual acuity may vary from minimal loss to hand movements, but loss of vision to light perception or no light perception is extremely rare. The visual acuity loss in the two eyes is usually quite symmetrical. Loss of color vision is a constant feature, and is usually more profound than the loss of visual acuity. Very early cases may present with isolated dyschromatopsia.

- Pupillary reactions are usually normal. The fundus may appear normal at first, though a careful examination may reveal nerve fiber layer losses in the papillomacular bundle. In the acute stages peripapillary dilated vessels and hemorrhages may be noted.
- The characteristic of this disorder is the visual field defect that consists of a centrocecal scotoma that begins nasal to the blind spot and extends to involve the fixation on both sides of the vertical meridian.
- Suspected toxicity can be confirmed through serum and urine analysis. 24-hours urine collection for heavy metal screening may also be helpful. In addition, serum vitamin levels may also be obtained. Associated systemic symptoms, such as parasthesia, ataxia, and hearing impairment may point towards the induced vitamin deficiencies.
- If the cause of the toxic neuropathy can be found, then discontinuation of its exposure in early stages can restore vision to near normal over several months.

BIBLIOGRAPHY

1. Solberg Y, Rosner M, Belkin M. The association between cigarette smoking and ocular diseases. Surv Ophthalmol. 1998;42(6):535-47. Review.
2. Kupersmith MJ, Weiss PA, Carr RE. The visual-evoked potential in tobacco-alcohol and nutritional amblyopia. Am J Ophthalmol. 1983;95(3):307-14.
3. Potts AM. Tobacco amblyopia. Surv Ophthalmol. 1973; 17(5):313-39. Review.
4. Foulds WS, Chisholm, Bronte-Stewart J, Reid HC. The investigation and therapy of the toxic amblyopias. Trans Ophthalmol Soc UK. 1970;90:739-63.
5. Friedmann AI. Visual field examination in the toxic and nutritional optic neuropathies. Trans Ophthalmol Soc UK. 1970;90:795-808.

CT AND MRI IN OPHTHALMOLOGY

COMPUTED TOMOGRAPHY
Indications
Ocular

- Injuries with suspected FB
- *Tumors:* Retinoblastoma.

Orbital Disease

- All proptosis
- Orbital fractures and trauma.

Neuro-ophthalmic Disease

Suspected intracranial tumors (e.g. unexplained optic atrophy, Foster-Kennedy syndrome, any hemianopia, especially a temporal loss, junctional scotoma, pediatric ocular motor nerve palsy).

Contraindications

- Pregnancy
- Contrast allergy (do only plain CT, or consider MRI).

Contrast not Required or Contraindicated in

- Contrast allergy
- Thyroid ophthalmopathy
- Orbital fractures and trauma.

MAGNETIC RESONANCE IMAGING
MRI is More Ueful than CT

Ocular disease: Malignant melanoma.
Orbital disease: Any apical lesions.
Neuro-ophthalmic disease:
- Cranial nerve palsy
- Multiple sclerosis
- Aneurysms

- AV fistulas
- Brainstem and posterior fossa.

MR OR CT ANGIOGRAPHY

Aneurysms, AV fistulas and malformations.

MRI Contraindicated

- Metallic implants—pacemakers, FBs, aneurysm clips (IOLs are not contraindications)
- Claustrophobic patients.

7

Vitreoretinal Diseases

- Prophylaxis Against Retinal Detachment
- Retinopathy of Prematurity
- Management of a Case of Scleral Fixated Intraocular Lens
- Heredomacular Dystrophy
- Fundus Fluorescein Angiography
- Evaluation and Preparation of Patient for Vitreoretinal Surgery
- Management of a Case of Vitreous Hemorrhage
- Vascular Disease—Artery and Vein Occlusion
- Diabetic Retinopathy
- Management of a Case of Macular Disorders—Macular Hole, Epiretinal Membrane and Vitreomacular Traction Syndrome
- Emergency Vitreoretinal Cases and Management of a Case of Intraocular Foreign Body
- Acquired Macular Disease—Central Serous Chorioretinopathy, Age-related Macular Degeneration
- Intravitreal Injections
- Retinoblastoma
- Acute Postoperative Endophthalmitis
- Outpatient Department Procedures—Ultrasound A and B Scan, Lasers and Cryotherapy

PROPHYLAXIS AGAINST RETINAL DETACHMENT

ABSOLUTE INDICATIONS

- Symptomatic retinal breaks
- Retinal tears in aphakic and pseudophakic eyes
- Retinal breaks in fellow eye when one eye had retinal detachment
- Retinal breaks in eyes with high myopia
- Lattice degeneration with atrophic holes and subclinical retinal detachment (less than 4 disc diameters)
- Traumatic retinal dialysis.

RELATIVE INDICATIONS

- Lattice degeneration with atrophic holes in the above circumstances
- Lattice degeneration in eyes undergoing LASIK procedure
- *Eyes with coloboma of choroid:*
  - Especially where treatment is safe, e.g. where the disc is not involved in the coloboma
  - Where there is intercalary membrane detachment
- Glaucomatous eyes where in pilocarpine treatment is contemplated.

RELATIVE CONTRAINDICATIONS

- Eyes with multiple rows of lattice degeneration 360 degrees, especially with very posterior lesions—the risk of treatment is also significant and the potential benefit questionable
- Eyes with coloboma with optic disc involved. Avoiding the disc area and treating the rest of the coloboma margin may not be of much prophylactic value and treating the disc area of the coloboma with laser in eyes with attached retina have risk of causing nerve fiber layer damage.

SPECIAL SITUATIONS

- *In the presence of significant cataract:* It is best that the cataract is removed and the lesions are treated approximately 3 to 4 weeks later. However, if there is urgent need to treat as in fresh horseshoe tears, etc. one can perform cryopexy.
- *Vitreous hemorrhage due to posterior vitreous detachment (PVD) where in retinal tear is not visualized:* Bed rest with head elevated position for a few days can facilitate enough clearance of the vitreous hemorrhage to permit identification of the retinal break which can be treated by cryopexy if laser is not possible.

TECHNIQUE OF TREATMENT

Laser Photocoagulation

- Preferred modality of treatment.
- Can be delivered by slit lamp or indirect ophthalmoscope.
- For peripheral lesions indirect ophthalmoscope with or without scleral indentation is preferred.
- Two to three rows of burns placed next to each other and around lesion.
- Anterior edge should also be well covered.
- At least the ora should be linked with the extreme ends of treatment if the entire anterior edge is not treated.
- Area of subretinal fluid should be surrounded.
- Supplemental cryo if laser is not possible for the entire lesion.
- Can space the treatment in more than one session if the treatment needed is extensive.
- If treatment is extensive, topical steroids can be given for 4 to 5 days, 3 to 4 times a day.
- The efficacy of treatment can be judged after 10 days if need be.

Cryopexy

- Preferred in cases with relatively hazy media (cataract, vitreous hemorrhage, corneal opacity, etc.) where laser is found to be difficult.

- It is preferrable to treat with laser to the extent possible and then only resort to cryo for the rest.
- Mostly done under peribulbar anesthesia. Subconjunctival xylocaine injection can also be sufficient in limited treatments.
- Confluent cryo applications of one row produced around the lesion.
- In case of cataract, one can avoid cryo and treat with laser after cataract surgery provided there is no urgency.
- Eye needs to be patched for 5 ot 6 hours, if peribulbar anesthesia is given.
- Analgesics can be given if needed.
- Topical steroids are prescribed for 4 to 5 days, 3 to 4 times a day.
- Reviewing the next day is optional.
- Efficacy of treatment can be judged after 10 days if need be.

Follow-up

- It is ideal that all treated eyes are reviewed in 10 days to check for the efficacy of treatment.
- *PVD induced retinal tears:* Since crops of new retinal breaks can occur due to progressive vitreous detachment, it is important to examine these eyes carefully at intervals. Initial re-examination can be after 10 days and then after 1 month and subsequently after 3 to 4 months. Beyond 6 months new break formation is very rare.

Counseling

Patient are instructed on symptoms for emergency attention such as sudden onset shower of black spots (not one or two floaters), sudden onset persistent flashes of light (not transient flashes), or a shadow in the field of vision.

Consensus on Lesions and Frequency of Treatment among Vitreous Surgeons

Type of lesion	Phakic eyes	Highly myopic eyes	RD-Fellow eyes	Aphakic or pseudophakic eyes	Prior to cataract surgery
Atrophic holes	Rarely	Rarely	Rarely	Rarely	Rarely
Operculated holes	No	Rarely	Rarely	Rarely	Rarely
Lattice degeneration with or without holes	No	Rarely	Yes	Rarely	Rarely
Horseshoe tears	Yes	Yes	Yes	Yes	Yes
Subclinical retinal detachment	Yes	Yes	Yes	Yes	Yes
Dialysis	Yes	Yes	Yes	Yes	Yes

RETINOPATHY OF PREMATURITY

Minimal Relevant History to be Recorded

- Gestation age (weeks at delivery)
- Chronological age (weeks after birth)
- Birth weight
- Whether any supplemental oxygen therapy given (Ventilator support)
- History of blood transfusions
- History of neonatal septicemia
- History of concurrent illnesses
- History of multiple births
- Previous treatment if any.

EXAMINATION

- Dilated fundus examination with indirect ophthalmoscopy with scleral depression 3 to 4 weeks after birth or before discharge from the neonatal unit which ever is earlier.
- Dilate with combination of phenylephrine 2.5 percent and tropicamide 1 percent instilled twice at ten minutes interval with simultaneous punctual occlusion.
- In lieu of ideal combination of phenylephrine 10 percent and tropicamide 1 percent as mentioned above, one can mix 1 cc of 10 percent phenylephrine with 3 cc of 1 percent tropicamide (both commonly available). This gives a combination of phenylephrine 2.5 percent and tropicamide 0.75 percent.
- Instill a drop of paracaine (topical anesthetic).
- Use Alfonso or other infant speculum for exposure.
- Scleral indentation is done with a Wire Vectis.
- A condensing lens of 20 D is used for comparison with standard photograph. 28 D/30 D lens may also be used.

Data Recording

- Use retinopathy of prematurity (ROP) data sheet (Refer Annexure 1).
- Examine the cornea and anterior chamber.
- Mention extent of pupillary dilation, presence of iris vascular engorgement, persistent pupillary membrane, vitreous haze or hemorrhage
- Record location of ROP—zone 1, zone 2 or zone 3.
- Enter number of clock hours involved.
- Note severity of the disease by stages 1 through 5.
- Look for signs of posterior plus disease (sufficient vascular dilatation and tortuosity present in at least 2 quadrants of the eye), A + symbol is added to the ROP stage number to designate the presence of plus disease. For example, stage 2 ROP combined with posterior vascular dilatation and tortuosity should be written "stage 2 +ROP".
  Plus disease is defined as a degree of dilation and tortuosity of the posterior retinal blood vessels as defined by a standard photograph.
- Look for signs of pre-plus disease and can be noted beside the stage, for example, "stage 2 with pre-plus disease".
  Pre-plus disease is defined as abnormal dilatation and tortuosity of the posterior pole vessels that are insufficient for the diagnosis of plus disease but that demonstrate more arterial tortuosity and more venous dilatation than normal.
- Look for signs of aggressive posterior retinopathy (AP-ROP).
- The AP-ROP posterior pole is defined as vascular dilation and tortuosity of all 4 quadrants that is out of proportion to the peripheral retinopathy most commonly in zone 1 causing inability to differentiate arterioles and venules.
- Notice previous treatment marks—cryo or laser scars, if any.
- Watch for apneic spells (crying is a good sign).

TREATMENT

- If normal retinal vascularization is seen 360 degrees up to ora serrata, only follow-up examination is needed perhaps at 6 months. It is assumed that 360 degrees examination could be performed adequately and normal vascularization was noted up to ora serrata. In case of any doubt a review after 1 week is advised.
- If retinal vasculature is immature and extends into zone 2 but no retinopathy is present, follow-up examination should be planned at 2 weeks. Either normalization takes place or ROP develops.
- If retinal vasculature is immature and extends into zone 1 but no retinopathy is present and there is no plus disease, weekly examination is mandatory. Sometimes, it can develop into aggressive posterior ROP (AP-ROP) which does not necessarily follow classical 1-3 staging.
- Stage 1 or 2 ROP in zone 2/3 with no plus disease, follow-up examination should be planned at 1 to 2 weeks.
- Stage 1 or 2 ROP in zone 1 or stage 3 ROP in zone 2, with no plus disease, follow-up examination should be planned at < 1 week .
- Refer Flow charts 7.1 and 7.2 for complete planning. *Type 1 ROP is defined as zone 1, any stage with plus disease, or zone 1, stage 3 without plus disease or zone 2,*

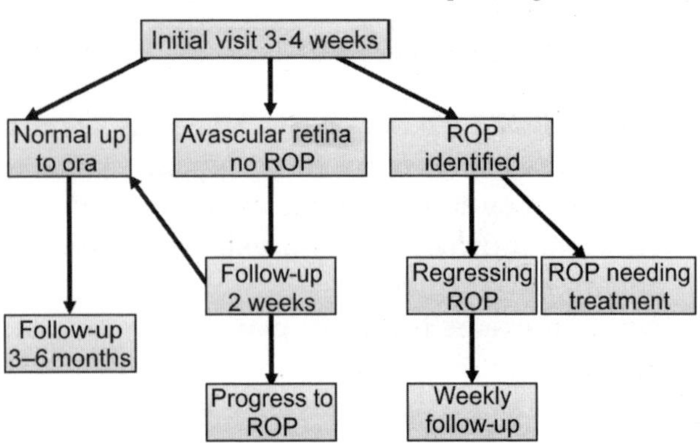

Flow chart 7.1: Treatment planning

Flow chart 7.2: Laser treatment planning

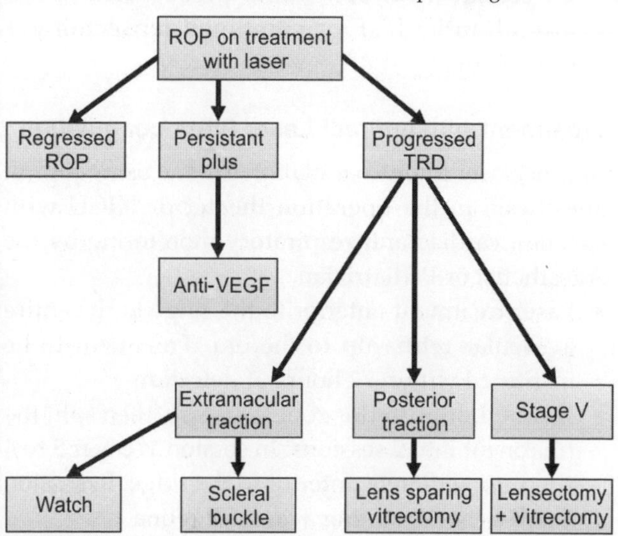

stage 2 or 3 with plus disease (type 1 includes eyes with threshold ROP).
**Type 2 ROP is defined as zone 1, stage 1 or 2 without plus disease or zone 2, stage 3 without plus disease.*

Indications for Laser Treatment

- Zone 1 ROP in any stage with plus disease will need laser treatment as described below within 72 hours of detection.
- Zone 1 ROP and stage 3 with no plus disease will need laser treatment as described below within 72 hours of detection.
- Zone 2 and stage 2 or 3 with plus disease will need laser treatment as described below within 72 hours of detection.
- Aggressive posterior retinopathy (AP-ROP) will need laser treatment as described below within 48 hours of detection.
- Stages 4 and 5 will require surgical repair of retinal detachment with scleral buckling, lens sparing

vitrectomy with or without preoperative intra-vitreal anti-VEGF or combined lensectomy + vitrectomy.

Treatment with Indirect Laser Photocoagulation

Indirect laser photocoagulation is done using topical anesthesia in the operation theater or NICU with constant cardiac and respiratory monitoring by the Anesthetist or Pediatrician.

- Laser treatment anterior to the ridge to the entire avascular retina up to the ora. Treatment to be instituted within 72 hours of detection.
- If zone 1 or posterior zone 2 disease, then split the treatment into 2 sessions. In session 1, cover 3 to 4 rows immediately anterior to the ridge. In session 2 cover the remaining avascular retina.
- Topical steroid with or without antibiotic is prescribed in q.i.d dosage for 5 days.

SURGICAL MANAGEMENT

Scleral Buckling in ROP

- Surgical repair of retinal detachment with scleral buckling done for stage 4a/4b/rare cases of stage 5
- Exoplant used is 240 band
- Scleral tunnels are made
- Placement of the band at site of highest ridge
- Indentation facilitated by paracentesis
- *Removal of buckle or band cutting:* Approximately at 1 year age to prevent erosion into developing eye.

Vitrectomy in ROP

- Lens sparing vitrectomy with or without preoperative intravitreal anti-VEGF or combined lensectomy + vitrectomy.
- Intravitreal anti-VEGF is given in half the adult dose (0.625 mg 0.75 mm to 1 mm from pars plana) if required after explaining the possible risk in

operation theater following sterile precautions under topical anesthesia.

**Currently anti-VEGF is used for failed laser therapy or prior to surgery in very florid disease rather than as primary treatment.*

Follow-up

- If initial fundus exam was normal and in cases with spontaneous regression of ROP as well as laser induced regression of ROP, repeat exam after 6 months is indicated to watch for myopia, strabismus, amblyopia.
- Watch for delayed complications like macular dragging, cataract, glaucoma or retinal detachment later on.
- If significant refractive error is present as mentioned below-correction of the same with glasses is mandatory:
  - Myopia of more than > – 4.00 D.
  - Hyperopia with no manifest deviation of > +6.00 D.
  - Hyperopia with esotropia > +2.00 D.
  - Astigmatism of > 3.00 Dcyl.
  - Any anisometropia of > +2.5 Dsp/> – 2.5 Dsp/ > 2.5 Dcyl.

Annexure: I

SANKARA NETHRALAYA

18, COLLEGE ROAD, CHENNAI – 600 006

ROP EVALUATION FORM

Patient Name ________________________________   MRD No. ________________

Gestational Age ________________   Birth Date ________________

Weight ________________   Exam Date ________________

ANTERIOR SEGMENT

	OD		OS	
iris rubeosis	yes	no	yes	no
corneal abnormality	yes	no	yes	no
suspect glaucoma	yes	no	yes	no

FUNDUS

Zone 3   Zone 2   Zone 1

	OD		OS	
vitreous hemorrhage	yes	no	yes	no
plus disease	yes	no	yes	no
prethreshold	yes	no	yes	no
(zone 1 any stage, zone 2 with stage 2+, zone 3 or zone 2 stage 3+ but not reaching threshold clock hours. Need to examine in one week)				
threshold	yes	no	yes	no
(zone 1 or zone 2 with stage 3+, 5 contiguous sectors or 8 composite sectors. Cryo + herapy within 72 hours)				

OD   Immaure, no ROP ________   Mature ________

ROP Higher stage ________   Lowest zone ________   Total number clock hours ________

OS   Immaure, no ROP ________   Mature ________

ROP Higher stage ________   Lowest zone ________   Total number clock hours ________

Re-examine in ________ weeks.

Physician's signature ________________

CPAPM 60.1/REV.0

MANAGEMENT OF A CASE OF SCLERAL FIXATED INTRAOCULAR LENS

INDICATIONS

- *Secondary intraocular lens (IOL) in aphakic eyes (previous ICCE/lensectomy):*
  - Intolerance to or frequent loss of contact lenses
  - Certain job profiles, contact lenses are not practical option
  - Inability to adjust to aphakic glasses
  - Unilateral aphakia.
- Intraocular lens exchange for subluxated/dislocated IOL
- Post-traumatic cataract with damage to the zonules/posterior capsule
- Subluxation/dislocation of natural crystalline lens
- Attempted cataract surgery with drop of nucleus or cortical remnants and loss of adequate capsular support
- Traumatic cataract with glaucoma for combination surgery with filtering procedures.

CONTRAINDICATIONS

- Systemic bleeding disorders (risk of intraoperative bleeding)
- Age below 4 years
- *Ocular conditions where scleral fixated IOL may be contraindicated:*
  - Infection
  - Retinal detachment
  - Microphthalmic eye with previous intracapsular cataract extraction (ICCE)
  - Rubeosis/Neovascular glaucoma (NVG)
  - Known cystoid macular edema (CME)
  - Endothelial decompensation (unless planning with PK)
  - Known recurrent uveitis

- Post-trauma; disorganized anterior segment with extensive scarring
- Very high myopia (IOL may not be needed)
- Megalocornea with sulcus diameter more than overall diameter of the IOL (relative contraindication, will need specially designed IOL).

PREOPERATIVE EVALUATION

- Vision and refraction
- Routine examination of eyes and adnexae
- *Specially look for:*
  - Mobility of the conjunctiva over probable location of fixation sutures
  - Corneal clarity/edema/scarring
  - Cataract section integrity
  - Anterior chamber inflammation
  - Iris and capsular integrity
  - Integrity of ciliary sulcus
  - IOL/crystalline lens (if present), its location/its mobility/fibrosis around it
- Fundus examination
- Status of retina/vitreous (including RD)
- CME/epiretinal membrane (ERM)
- Peripheral retinal lesions
- Vitreous traction
- Diabetic retinopathy (DBR)
- To check patency of nasolacrimal passage.

TIMINGS OF SURGERY

- Elective surgery
- *Dislocations during primary cataract surgery:*
  - Repositioning/scleral fixation at the same sitting
  - After 2-3 weeks, if:
    - ◆ Vitrectomy facilities are not available
    - ◆ Surgeon is not experienced with vitrectomy techniques

TECHNIQUES

- Internal suturing (e.g. Lasso), possible only for dislocated IOL
- *Scleral fixated intraocular lens (SFIOL) with intrascleral knot:*
  - Scleral flaps preferred
  - Radial keratotomy (RK) marks used for meridian selection
  - 10-0 Prolene tied around haptic, eyelet at one end and intrascleral at the other end
  - Knot under scleral flap.

HEREDOMACULAR DYSTROPHY

HISTORY

- What is the duration of dimness of vision?
- Is the dimness of vision slowly progressive?
- Is there any associated decrease in side vision?
- Is there any associated difficulty in night vision?
- Is there any associated photo aversion or difficulty in bright light?
- Is there history of consanguinity amongst parents?
- Is any other family member affected? If yes, their details if available.
- Is there any history of long-term medications—especially chloroquine, desferroxamine, thioridazine.
- Are any previous records/photographs/investigations reports available?
- Are there any other systemic abnormalities?

EXAMINATION

- *Best corrected visual acuity:* To spend more time with the patient to try to make him/her read the maximum possible
- *Slit-lamp exam:* Look for any corneal crystals, whorls and any significant
- *Lens changes:*
  - Intraocular pressure (IOP)
  - Fundus
- Indirect ophthalmoscopy and + 78 D examination
- *Disc:* Look for any pallor
- *Arteries:* Look for attenuation
- Describe in details the macular lesion—use terms like discrete atrophic lesion, ill defined atrophic lesion, tapetal sheen, annular atrophic ring, bull's eye
- Maculopathy, discrete/atrophic/coalesced flecks, etc.

- Describe the exact location of the macular lesion
- Make a precise drawing
- Note if the foveal center is involved
- Look for any flecks at the posterior pole
- Look for any retinal deposits/crystals at the posterior pole
- Look for any evidence of choroidal neovascular membrane (CNVM)
- Examine the retinal periphery–specifically mention if the retinal lustre is normal or abnormal or if any pigmentary changes is present.

INVESTIGATIONS

- *At first visit:*
  - Electroretinogram (ERG), multifocal ERG
  - Electro-oculography (EOG)—if Best's dystrophy is suspected
  - Color vision–FM–100 Hue Test–if the near vision is > N 18
  - Fundus photograph
  - Fundus fluorescein angiography (FFA).
- *Visual fields:* Preferably the same program should be repeated in future
- *At subsequent visits:*
  - Fundus photo
  - ERG, multifocal ERG—at consultant's discretion— usually once in 2-years
  - FFA—at consultant's discretion
- *Treatment:*
  - Glass prescription
  - Low visual aids
  - Tinted glasses for cone dystrophy patients— refer patient to LVA
  - Department for the same
  - Advice ocular examination of other family members
  - Genetic counseling

- Do not give a very poor prognosis to the patients, emphasize on the positive side - the patient is very unlikely to be completely blind
- They usually retain enough peripheral vision to be able to do day-to-day activities on their own
- Home Amslers to detect CNVM in case of Best's disease.

RETINITIS PIGMENTOSA

History

- Age of onset of symptoms
- Duration of night blindness
- Duration of progressive loss of visual fields
- Duration of dimness of vision. Is it progressive?
- Family history of RP. If yes, were they examined at SN? If yes their MRD numbers
- History of trauma
- History of drug intake
- History of hearing disorder, ataxia, nystagmus.
- History of mental retardation
- History of heart disease
- History of hypogenitalism, obesity, polydactyly
- History of diarrhea, skeletal deformities.

EXAMINATION

- Best corrected visual acuity
- *Slit-lamp examination:* Look for PSC cataract, keratoconus.
- IOP
- Fundus examination
- I/O and +78 D
- Disc pallor
- Arteriolar attenuation
- RPE mottling, granularity
- *Pigmentary changes:* Fine/Clumps
- *Location:* Central, midperipheral, perivascular
- Peripheral lipid exudation
- Presence of tapetal reflex/metallic sheen

- Presence of any macular lesion
- *Vitreous Abnormalities:* Pigments, vitreous condensation, PVD.

INVESTIGATIONS

- *At first visit:*
  - ERG
  - *Visual fields:* Preferably the same program should be repeated in future
  - *Fundus photograph:* Consultant's discretion
  - *FFA:* Consultant's discretion. It can be ordered in atypical cases or in cases in which the diagnosis is not very apparent.

- *At subsequent visits:*
  - *Fundus photo:* Consultant's discretion
  - *ERG:* Can be repeated once in 2 years (if previous. recordable wave amplitudes)
  - *Visual fields:* Can be repeated once in 2 years.

TREATMENT

- Glass prescription
- Low visual aids
- Field expanders
- Cataract surgery if required
- Treatment of cystoid macular edema with acetazolamide
- Advice ocular examination of other family members
- Address other associated systemic problems
- Genetic counseling
- Rehabilitation
- Information regarding any new scientific development.

FUNDUS FLUORESCEIN ANGIOGRAPHY

INDICATIONS
- Diabetic retinopathy
- CRVO, BRVO
- CRAO, BRAO
- CNVM- Other causes
- Parafoveal telangiectasis
- CSR
- Cystoid macular edema
- Retinal artery microaneurysm
- Hypertensive retinopathy
- Heredomacular dystrophies
- Exudative retinal detachment
- *Vascular ocular tumors:* Angioma, choroidal hemangioma
- *Inflammatory disorders:* APMPPE, GHPC, MEWDS, VKH, etc.

CONTRAINDICATIONS
Absolute contraindication: Allergy to fluorescein

Relative contraindication
- Pregnancy
- Lactating mothers
- Diabetic nephropathy
- Chronic renal failure
- Mental retardation
- Pediatric age group
- *Ocular:* Media opacity that would prevent a proper evaluation.

PREINJECTION INSTRUCTIONS
- Fasting 2 hours prior to the test
- Informed consent form to be signed
- Patient to be explained regarding the procedure
- Inform about nausea.

PROCEDURE

- Check FFA form for diagnosis, area of interest to be photographed and for any specific instructions
- To check if routine or digital imaging has been asked for
- To check if fundus photo (montage) along with FFA is required
- To check case sheet and FFA form for the eye to be investigated
- Ensure pupil is fully dilated
- Patient seated in front of the camera and explained the procedure
- Adjust camera in relation to patient's eye
- Fixate eye using a fixation target
- IV scalp vein placed by the nurse and its patency ensured with universal precaution
- Avoid extravasation
- Stereoscopic red-free photographs are taken in each eye prior to the injection of the fluorescein dye
- Choose correct field size based upon pathology to be evaluated
- Timer to be started at the start of the injection of fluorescein dye
- Fluorescein is injected rapidly (less than 5 seconds if possible)
- Photographs to be taken 8 to 10 seconds after commencement of dye injection
- To take standard magnification photograph of the macula in all the cases
- In cases of repeat digital angiograms, to ensure that the name of the patient is entered in the same way as the previous visits
- If separate runs are required for the two eyes, then the other eye FFA can be scheduled the next day
- However, it is possible to take early pictures at the same sitting in case of most bilateral lesions
- Sequence of fields of the fundus in case of bilateral conditions is to start with disc with macula, go clockwise in periphery, come back to disc and macula switch to fellow eye repeat the same, come back to disc and macula.

POSTINJECTION INSTRUCTIONS

- Discoloration of urine for 24 to 48 hour
- Discoloration of vision
- Discoloration of skin for 6 to 12 hours
- Temporary discontinuation of breastfeeding in lactating mothers

ICG ANGIOGRAPHY

Indications

- ARMD subtype retinal angiomatous proliferation (RAP)
- Polypoidal choroidal vasculopathy
- Rare—inflammatory disorders, e.g. MEWDS, APMPPE
- Any threatening macular lesions not picked up by FFA.

Contraindications

- Allergy to ICG dye
- Allergy to any iodine compounds, seafood.

Relative Contraindications

- Pregnancy, lactation
- Poor systemic condition of the patient.

Preangiogram Instructions

To be fasting for 2 hours before procedure.

Procedure

- To check requisition form. Check diagnosis, area of interest any specific instructions, eye to be photographed
- Check file to see eye to be examined
- Informed consent form to be signed
- Dilate pupils
- Explain procedure to the patient
- Inject 2 ml of aqueous solvent provided with the ICG into the ICG vial. Dissolve it by shaking. Load

into a syringe. Load 5 ml of normal saline into another syringe.

- Explain the procedure to the patient
- Start the scalp vein set. The photographer has to adjust the camera and inform the nurse to start the infusion. Inject the dye quickly, immediately followed by the normal saline. The photographs are then taken at every 15 second interval. The late phase photograph is taken 20 minutes later.

** If both ICG and FFA are required, then ICG is first performed and FFA done while waiting for the late films of ICG.*

**If separate runs of ICG are required for each eye, then the angiogram for the other eye is done the next day.*

EMERGENCY EQUIPMENT NEEDED IN FFA ROOM

- Emesis basin
- Oxygen
- Spygmomanometer and stethoscope
- Couch for patient to lie down
- Ice pack
- Tourniquet
- Disposable needles
- Disposable syringes
- IV set and scalp vein set
- Airway device
- Oxygen cylinder
- Ambu bag
- Inj Adrenaline
- Inj Atropine
- Inj Avil
- Inj Betnesol
- Inj Decadron
- Inj Deriphylline
- Inj Dextrose 5%
- Inj Dextrose 25%
- Inj Dextrose 50%

- Inj Ephedrine
- Inj Fortwin
- Inj Lasix
- Inj Potassium chloride
- Inj Sodium bicarbonate
- Inj Sodium chloride
- Inj Stemetil.

MULTIFOCAL ELECTRORETINOGRAM

Indications

- To distinguish retinal diseases from optic nerve disease
- Details of extent of lesion
- Sensitive indicator for retinal drug toxicity
- Postoperative assessment following V-R surgery
- Assess subclinical retinal changes in diabetic retinopathy.

Not possible to do test in
- Poor fixation
- Poor vision
- Uncooperative patients
- Dense media opacity
- Nystagmus.

Procedure

Electrode Placement

- Bipolar Burian Allen electrodes or DTL electrodes are used for multifocal electroretinogram (mfERG) recordings with a gold cup electrode attached to the earlobe as a ground electrode.
- Using the same electrodes and amplifiers employed for standard full field ERG recording, a single continuous ERG record is obtained. The subject fixates on the central elements of stimulus, usually aided by a cross or marker. Recordings are done monocularly.

Stimulus Parameters

- The multifocal stimulus is displayed on a CRT monitor or on a LED displays. The display contains an array of hexagons; the most commonly used displays contain 61 or 103 hexagons. The scaling of hexagons is determined by photoreceptor topography across the retina and is scaled to produce local responses of approximately equal amplitude. Central hexagons are smaller than the peripheral hexagons. During stimulation, the display flickers because each hexagon goes through a pseudorandom binary m-sequence of black and white presentations. Each hexagon has a probability of 0.5 being white or black on each frame change. Typically, the frame is changed every 13.33 ms (a frame rate of 75 Hz).
- Normal room lighting is used during mfERG recording. At the viewing distance of 53 cm, the hexagonal stimulus subtends approximately 35 degrees horizontally and 31 degrees vertically. The high and low luminance levels of the stimulus are about 128 cd/m^2 and 3 cd/m^2. A Grass Amplifier (15LT) with band pass from 10-300 Hz and gain of 50,000 is used to record mfERG. The stimulus pattern comprises of a central hexagon corresponding to the fovea and five concentric rings at different eccentricities corresponding to the para macular region. Ring 1 (R1) subtended 1.6 degree in diameter, ring 2 (R2) 1.6 to 6 degree, ring 3 (R3) 6 to 11.4 degree, ring 4 (R4) 11.4 to 18.2 degree, ring 5 (R5) 18.2 to 26.2 degree and ring 6 (R6) 26.2 to 35 degree. Parameters measured in mfERG are amplitudes and implicit times.

CLINICAL PROTOCOL

Preparation of the Patient

The pupils are fully dilated before the mfERG recordings. Patient is made to sit comfortably in front of the CRT monitor. Good fixation is essential. Fixation is monitored throughout. Refractive error of the patient is corrected with the help of inbuilt refractor to maintain good retinal image quality.

REPORTING
Mode of Display

Trace arrays: These show topographic variations and demonstrate the quality of the records.

Group averages: Arranging responses by groups is useful to define regions with fundus pathology.

Three-dimensional plots: The 3-D plots, without accompanying trace arrays, can be misleading.

The first-order kernel responses are taken for interpretation. The trace array represents ERG responses for each hexagon. The N1 response amplitude is measured from the starting baseline to the base of the N1 trough; the P1 response amplitude is measured from the N1 trough to the P1 peak. The peak times (implicit times) of N1 and P1 are measured from the stimulus onset. Measurements of group averages should routinely include the N1 and P1 amplitudes and peak times.Ring responses represent mfERG responses summed by rings and expressed in nV/deg^2.

MULTIFOCAL VISUAL EVOKED POTENTIAL
Indications

- Optic neuritis
- Ischemic optic neuropathy
- Compressive optic neuropathy
- Assess the topography of the visual field defect
- Children who do not respond to HVF 30 -2 testing
- Unreliable visual field report
- To differentiate visual field of retinal diseases using mfERG from the optic nerve diseases using multifocal visual evoked potential (mfVEP).

Not Possible to do Test in

- Poor fixation
- Uncooperative patients
- Dense media opacity
- Nystagmus eyes.

Procedure

Basic Technology

Till date there is no standard protocol recommended by International Society for Clinical Electrophysiology of Vision Standard (ISCEV) for performing mfVEP.

Electrode Placement

Gold disc surface electrodes are used to record mfVEP. Active electrodes are placed 4 cm above the inion and 4 cm lateral to and 1 cm above the inion on either side which are referred to as midline and lateral channel respectively. The reference electrode is placed on the inion. The ground electrode is placed on the forehead (*Hood and Greenstein, 2003*).

Stimulus Parameters

The stimulus of multifocal VEP is termed as Dartboard pattern which contains 60 sectors. It subtends 44.5 degrees of visual diameter when viewed at 32 cm from the monitor (*Hood and Greenstein, 2003*). Each sector contains 16 checks of which 8 are black and 8 are white. The stimulus checks are scaled based on cortical magnification factor. The black and white checks in each sector reverses independently according to a pseudo random sequence known as a binary m-sequence. The responses are mathematically extracted by cross correlating the continuous VEP signal with the stimulus sequence during real time recording. The stimulus is delivered by cathode ray tube monitor at a frame rate of 75 Hz. The luminance of 100-200 cd/m^2 is used for white checks and less than 1 cd/m^2 is used for black checks. The band pass filter is set between 3 and 100 Hz.

Clinical Protocol

Preparation of the Patient

Subject should sit comfortably to minimize muscle artifacts during testing. The room light should be on with illumination ideal to the stimulus luminance. Monocular stimulation should be performed. The procedure should be done in the undilated pupil. Any abnormal pupil size should be noted. The fixation of the patient is monitored with a camera unit in instrument setting. The patient should be refracted.

Reporting

The interpretation of mfVEP response should include about latency and amplitude. Amplitude measurements are made between peaks and troughs of the deflections. Peak latency measurements should be taken from the onset of the stimulus to the peak of the component concerned.

The typical mfVEP waveform is a biphasic wave which is extracted from the first slice of second order kernel. It consists of negative and positive waves namely C1 and C2. The responses are also reversed in polarity along the horizontal meridian since the cells generating the responses in the visual cortex are oriented in opposite direction (*Baseler et al, 1994; Hood and Greenstein, 2003*).

ELECTRORETINOGRAM

Indications

- Heredomacular dystrophies like cone dystrophy, Stargardt's disease, Best's disease
- Retinitis pigmentosa (RP) and its variants
- Stationary and progressive night blindness—congenital stationary night blindness, Oguchi's disease, Fundus albipunctatus, etc.
- Gyrate atrophy
- Choroiderimia
- Foveal schisis

- Central retinal vein occlusion
- Vitamin A deficiency
- Ocular retinal siderosis
- Retinal drug toxicity
- Unexplained visual loss.

Contraindications

- External ocular infections/inflammation, e.g. conjunctivitis, severe blepharitis, corneal ulcers
- Corneal epithelial defects
- Recent postoperative cases.

Not Recommended in
Patients with nystagmus.

Indications for ERG Under General Anesthesia

In children not co-operative for ERG with topical anesthesia, in whom an ERG test is essential to establish the diagnosis.

Procedure

The Standards for Clinical Electroretinography published in 2008 by International Society for Clinical Electrophysiology of Vision (ISCEV) is followed for ERG recording.

Basic Technology

- *Electrodes:* A Burien-Allen electrode, incorporating both the active and the reference electrode to be used. Ground electrode to be placed at the earlobe.
- *Stimulus:* Fullfield Ganzfeld bowl is used for stimulating the mass retinal response. The standard stimulus strength of 3 cd/m^2 is used as a standard flash intensity. A standard background luminance of 30 cd/m^2 is used for light adaptation.
- The band pass of the amplifier should be set between the ranges of 0.3 to 300 Hz and be adjustable. The input impedance of the preamplifiers should be at least 10 M Ohm.

Clinical Protocol

The pupils are maximally dilated and the size of the pupil is noted. Dark adaptation is provided for at least 20 minutes. If either a fundus photograph or a FFA has been done prior to ERG testing on the same day, then the patient should be dark adapted for 1 hour. The electrodes are placed under dim red light during ERG recording.

The suggested protocol as per ISCEV standards are as follows:

- *Single flash rod response* is the first signal measured after dark adaptation. A dim white flash of 0.01 cd/m^2 is used presented at an interval of 2 seconds between flashes.
- *Maximal response or combined rod-cone response* is the second protocol in scotopic response. The standard flash of 3 cd/m^2 stimulated at an interval of at least 10 seconds between flashes.
- *Oscillatory potentials* is the third protocol recorded in scotopic condition. It is recorded using the same standard flash. High pass filter is set to 75-100 Hz and the low pass filter set at 300 Hz or above. Flash should be given 15 seconds apart.
- *Single flash cone response* is recorded after 10 minutes of light adaptation with a background luminance of 30 cd/m^2. It is recorded with standard flash with an interval of 0.5 seconds between flashes.
- *30 Hz flicker response* is recorded with standard flash presented 30 stimuli per second.

Reporting

The important components of ERG are:
- *a-wave:* Represents the negative deflection originates from photoreceptors.
- *b-wave:* Positive deflection following the initial negative a-wave which arises from bipolar and muller cells.

The amplitude and implicit time (time to peak) of a-wave and b-wave should be measured. The a-wave amplitude is measured from baseline of waveform to trough of a-wave; the b-wave amplitude is measured from a-wave trough to b-wave peak. The a-wave and b-wave implicit times are measured from the time of the flash to the peak of the wave. The protocols and its components are listed below:

- *Single flash rod response:* b-wave amplitude and implicit time is measured. The a-wave is absent.
- *Combined response:* Both a-wave and b-wave implicit times and amplitudes are measured.
- *Oscillatory potentials:* Either the presence or absence or reduction is observed.
- *Single flash cone response:* Both a-wave and b-wave implicit times and amplitudes are measured.
- *30 Hz flicker:* b-wave amplitude and implicit time is measured.

ELECTRO-OCULOGRAM

Indications

- Best's vitelliform macular dystrophy
- Adult vitelliform macular dystrophy.

Not possible to do test in
- Uncooperative patients
- Patients with nystagmus
- Poor fixation.

Procedure

The Standards for Clinical Electro-oculography published in 2006 by ISCEV to be followed.

Basic Technology

Electrodes: Four skin electrodes are placed on medial and lateral canthi of both eyes. Amplifier should be set between 0.1 to 30 Hz.

Clinical Protocol

Pupils are dilated before examination. During the test patients are instructed to make horizontal eye movements between fixation targets separated by 30 degrees in a rhythmic manner. Saccadic responses are recorded for 10 seconds in an every minute. EOG recording involves two phases namely:

1. *Dark phase:* Prior to the test, patients should be pre-adapted to ordinary room lighting for at least 15 minutes. The room lights are turned off and recordings made for 15 minutes in the dark. The minimum amplitude during this period is termed the dark trough. It usually occurs around 15 minutes.
2. *Light phase:* The light is then turned on and recording continued until the signal amplitude reaches a clearly defined peak, the light peak.

Reporting

Arden's ratio is calculated to interpret EOG report. It is the ratio of light peak to dark trough. The ratio of light peak to dark trough is measured.

VISUAL EVOKED POTENTIAL

Indications

- Optic neuritis/Demyelination
- Compressive optic neuropathy
- Ischemic optic neuropathy
- Assess the visual status objectively
- Visual integrity in media opacities
- Malingering subjects
- Assess infant's visual acuity
- To assess the drug induced optic neuropathy
- Assess the postoperative prognosis in vitreous hemorrhage.

Not possible to do test in
Uncooperative subjects.

Procedure

Basic Technology

As per ISCEV 2009 update, visual evoked potential (VEP) is recorded.

Electrode placement: The gold cup or silver electrodes are used to record VEP. The active electrode is placed 4 cm above the inion over the scalp. Reference electrode is placed on midline of the body over the scalp. The reference electrode is placed on the forehead.

Stimulus parameters: Two types of stimulus are commonly used: flash and pattern reversal.
1. *Flash VEP:* The flash VEP to be elicited by a standard flash of 3 cd/m^2 in Ganzfeld stimulator.
2. *Pattern reversal VEP:* The pattern stimulus consists of black and white checks that alternate from black to white or white to black. The mean lamination of the screen should be uniform. The reversal rate of alteration of pattern should be between 1 and 3 reversals per second or 0.5 to 1.5 Hz. It is performed with different checker sizes where smaller checker size stimulates foveal region and larger checker size stimulates parafoveal region. The pattern checker size should subtend 1 degree and 15 minute. The visual field should subtend atleast 15 degrees as per ISCEV standards.

Clinical Protocol

Preparation of the Patient

The VEP is recorded monocularly in undilated pupil. Patient has to be seated comfortably to minimize muscle artifact. Proper refractive correction should be in place. Fixation should be monitored through the test. Care should be taken to ensure that nonrecorded eye is patched properly while testing the stimulated eye.

Reporting

The latency (in ms) and amplitude (in μV) is measured in VEP waveforms. The amplitude is measured from trough to peak of the wave. Peak latency is measured from onset of the stimulus to the peak of the component.

- *Flash VEP* consists of N2 and P2 components, which occur at around 90 and 120 msec respectively. The amplitude and latency of P2 component is interpreted in flash VEP.
- *Pattern reversal VEP* consists of an N1 component around 75 ms, P1 component around 100 ms and N2 component around 135 ms. The latency and amplitude of P1 component for different checker sizes are interpreted in pattern reversal VEP.

OPTICAL COHERENCE TOMOGRAPHY FOR MACULAR DISEASES

This is an optical analog of ultrasound where instead of sound, infrared light is used to image the layers of the retina. Based on the reflectivity of the tissues, a false color code is assigned for interpretation. It is based on the principle of Michelson low coherence interferometry.

When to Order

- CME
- VMT
- ARMD
- CSR and PED
- Macular hole
- ERM
- Foveal cysts; pseudohole
- Diabetic CSME and macular edema due to other causes
- Optic pit
- Parafoveal telangiectasis
- In case of RD, when in doubt regarding the macular involvement.

When to Avoid

Media opacities:
- Moderate-to-dense cataract
- Vitreous hemorrhage
- PCO.

Bilaterally poor vision (poor fixation portion will not allow accurate scan placement).

Type of Scan Protocols

- *Fast macular scans/radial scans:* Useful in all cases of macular edema and can be used to map the retinal thickness and notice see the change on subsequent follow-up.

  Low resolution scans are used for screening purposes while high resolution scans are used for discerning the pathology.
- *Line scan:* Useful in visible discrete lesion like pigment epithelial detachment:ARMD:Scar:IPCV. Shows a lot more detail because of higher resolution.
- *Raster lines/cross hair:* It can be used in visible discrete lesion also.

Recommendation

A fast macular scar should always be done along with other scan since it helps us to map and follow-up the macular pathology over time.

Analyses

- *Retinal map:* Useful for all cases of macular edema.

  It can be generated only be fast macular scan; radial axis.
- *Retinal thickness:* This can be used for any scan protocol and only analyses the thickness for the individual scans.

  Demonstrated in 9 quadrants around the macula.

Procedure to be Followed for Every Patient

Always check for adequate pupillary dilation in order to avoid artefacts.

- *Data entry:* Enter the patients name, MRD No. and the diagnosis along with data for all the dialog boxes present. Helps in comparison with previous OCT scans and archiving.
- *Scanning:* All the scans should be optimized for Z offset and polarization before being acquisition.
- Poor quality images (sound/noises ratio of < 30 need not be considered good and reliable.
- The correct analysis protocols need to be matched with the correct scan protocols. (e.g. retinal map - fast macular scan).

Precautions

- This is a noncontact technique hence make sure that the lens is not touching the eye or eyelashes.
- Do not save unnecessary images as they fills up the hard disc space and the DVD ROM. Select the images; which give the maximum information.
- Always keep the lens of the patient module covered when not in use. This helps to avoid dust and moisture from degrading the lens and the quality of image.

EVALUATION AND PREPARATION OF PATIENT FOR VITREORETINAL SURGERY

HISTORY

- Duration of visual loss
- History of flashes, floaters-which quadrant
- History of of trauma
- History of previous ocular surgery-details of the same. If previous RD surgery has been done, to get detail of the same especially surgical drawings and buckle placement.
- Previous refractive error.

EXAMINATION

- Best corrected visual acuity
- PL recheck with indirect ophthalmoscopy in darkened room
- *Slit-lamp examination:* Look for corneal, iris, lens, sclera status and specifically exposed buckle/suture in patients with history of previous buckle surgery
- Applanation tonometry
- Indirect ophthalmoscopy
- Extent of RD
- Location of retinal breaks
- Macula involvement, additional macular pathology
- Posterior extent of the breaks
- Whether old/fresh RD
- Vitreous changes—haze, hemorrhage
- PVD status
- Dislocated lens/IOL
- Any associated choroidal detachment
- Fellow eye assessment
- Ultrasound in hazy media mainly for retinal status, choroidal detachment and PVD assessment

- OCT for macular status in macular hole, epiretinal membrane
- VEP mainly for evaluation of salvage ability of traumatized eyes, and in children.

DISCUSSION WITH PATIENT

- Explain nature of disease to the patient-use drawings, models if necessary
- Explain the treatment options available
- Explain in brief regarding the surgical procedure
- Explain prognosis to the patient
- Explain regarding anatomical and functional outcomes
- Explain possibility of recurrence and need for re-surgery
- Explain need for any particular head position to be maintained after surgery
- Explain regarding anesthesia, duration of surgery, postoperative status, hospital stay required, restrictions to be followed in postoperative period.
- Explain need for patient to undergo blood investigations and physician check-up prior to surgery to get physician clearance for surgical intervention
- Patients with macula attached RD or RD with recently detached macula or fresh giant retinal tear should be admitted on the same day for early surgery.

PREOPERATIVE PREPARATION

- *Check case sheet for laboratory investigations:*
    - Hb, TLC, DLC, platelet count
    - Random blood sugar (Postprandial blood sugar if patient is a diabetic)
    - HIV testing, HB_SAg, HCV, Optional Non-treponemal (RPR), Treponemal (TPHA) in serum
- Urine–routine evaluation

- X-ray chest–if surgery is under general anesthesia and patient is above 40 years or if the surgery under steroid cover
- ECG–if patient is above 40 years
- Physician clearance for local or general anesthesia
- Preoperative retinal drawing
- Preoperative instructions to be given
- Preoperative antibiotic drops.

ROLE OF CONSULTANT AND VITREORETINAL ASSISTANT

- Admission orders to be written
- Check perception of light, eye to be operated
- Check for any ocular/systemic infective focus
- Check case sheet–diagnosis, allergies, eye to be operated, laboratory investigations, physician clearance, previous surgery notes
- Check consent forms
- DBR values if required
- Fill preoperative order sheet
- Mention eye to be operated, type of anesthesia, preoperative medication, preoperative dilatation orders, time of surgery, drug sensitivity.
- Detailed large drawing–in all cases in which some details of the retina is visualized, in all cases requiring a scleral buckle procedure
- Other eye drawing to be done–large drawing in case any procedure is to be done in the other eye
- Check if any ocular prosthesis is present on the other side. If present, it has to be removed and antibiotic drops instilled in the socket
- Give detailed preoperative instructions to the patient regarding time of the surgery, fasting and bathing
- Time of surgery
- Preoperative fasting instructions
- To remain fasting for 6 hours prior to surgery if surgery under general or 2 hours if under local anesthesia, except for babies getting breast milk, fasting time is 4 hours

- Instructions to wash face with soap and water on the evening prior to the surgery and in the morning on the day of surgery
- To have head bath in the morning on the day of surgery
- Instructions for an adult attendant to be present with the patient at least 2 hours prior to the surgery and until surgery is completed
- Explain any preoperative positioning if required.

PREOPERATIVE MEASURES IN DIABETIC PATIENTS

- Diabetic patients are usually admitted following diabetic control and fitness from physician, unless it is an emergency
- On admission
- Check previous blood sugar reports
- Check medicines advised by physician and verify with patient if it is being taken properly
- Ensure that the ward nurse has tested the patients urine for sugar and ketones
- Preoperative orders (in addition to usual orders)
- Continue all medications as advised on the day previous and day after the surgery
- Stop all diabetic medicines on the day of surgery
- Fasting period as in normal patients but to ensure it does not get unduly extended
- Monitoring and treatment of diabetes on day of surgery
- Blood sugar is estimated 3 times on the day by ward nurse (fasting, 1 pm and 8 pm) and this is informed to the physician and diabetic medicines are given as advised
- Blood sugar is estimated if advised by the physician or in case of suspected hypoglycemia
- Urine sugar and ketone bodies charting maintained
- Blood sugar control on the day of surgery with plain insulin.

PREOPERATIVE MEASURES IN HIGH-RISK CASES

- Ensure that the high-risk has been clearly explained to the patient by the physician and the operating consultant
- Ensure that the high-risk consent form duly filled is in the file
- See that proper physician clearance has been obtained and the reports of the investigations done are available in the file.

GUIDELINES FOR PATIENT COUNSELING IN VITREORETINAL SURGICAL CASES

For Simple Scleral Buckle Surgery

Factors Indicating Poor Anatomical Outcome

- Preoperative choroidal detachment
- Preoperative vitreous haze
- Early proliferative vitreoretinopathy (PVR) changes
- Total retinal detachment (RD)
- Macula detached RD
- Relatively posterior retinal breaks
- Retinal breaks in multiple quadrants
- Old age of the patient
- Unhealthy underlying RPE
- Fellow eye had developed recurrent RD due to PVR
- Factors indicating poor visual outcome
- Macula 'off' RD
- Long-standing RD
- Unhealthy underlying RPE at the macula
- Presence of macular hole, ERM
- Disc pallor, cupping.

Retinal Detachment with Proliferative Vitreoretinopathy Cases

- Long-standing disease
- Severe hypotony, choroidal detachment, vitreous haze
- Severe PVR, Inferior retinal breaks, Stiff retina, extensive subretinal gliosis, macular hole with RD
- High myopic eyes

Trauma Cases

- History of penetrating injury especially with posterior scleral tears, vitreous loss, IOFB
- Presence of rubeosis, complicated cataract, thick membrane in pupillary area, cyclitic membranes, extensive peripheral anterior synechiae
- Ultrasound test showing extensive taut vitreous membranes, vitreous incarceration, subretinal hemorrhage, choroidal hemorrhage, reduced axial length, choroidal thicknening, poor corneal status.

Diabetic Cases

- Tractional retinal detachment (TRD) involving macula, table-top TRD
- Extensive vascular proliferation
- Combined RD
- Absence of PVD on ultrasound, especially in diabetic vitreous hemorrhage with TRD cases
- Presence of rubeosis, angle NV
- Cases of recurrent vitreous hemorrhage showing anterior hyaloid proliferation.

Definitions

- *Anatomical success:* Refers to attached retina with clear media
- *Functional success:* Refers to expected visual improvement following anatomical success.

MANAGEMENT OF A CASE OF VITREOUS HEMORRHAGE

HISTORY

- Duration of visual loss
- History of trauma
- History of flashes floaters prior to visual loss
- History of diabetes mellitus (DM), hypertension (HTN)
- History of any bleeding disorders
- History of similar episode in the past
- History of similar complaints in the fellow eye
- History of head injury (Terson's syndrome).

EXAMINATION

- Best corrected visual acuity (BCVA)
- Slit-lamp–check for rubeosis before dilatation, lens status, uveitis
- IOP check
- Gonioscopy–to rule out angle NV in cases suspected of having central retinal vein occlusion (CRVO).

INDIRECT OPHTHALMOSCOPY

- Vitreous hemorrhage–fresh/old
- Intragel/Subhyaloid/Preretinal hemorrhage/ Subretinal hemorrhage
- Any fibrovascular proliferation seen
- If any retinal details seen
- If retinal periphery visualized
- If disc is seen hazily
- If any retinal vasculitis seen
- Any mass lesion
- I/O with indentation
- If there is a strong suspicion of retinal break being the cause of vitreous hemorrhage
- No proliferative disorder suspected

- Gentle indentation with slow release of the pressure during indentation
- Fellow eye examination–evidence of Eales disease, Pars planitis, diabetic retinopathy, HT retinopathy, BRVO, CRVO, ARMD, IPCV.

INVESTIGATIONS

Ultrasound

- Vitreous echoes intragel/retrohyaloid
- *PVD status:* Complete, incomplete, points of attachment, mobility
- *Any associated TRD:* Its location
- *Macular status:* TRD, pre/subretinal haem, disciform scar
- Mass lesion
- Retinal breaks.

Ultrasound Biomicroscopy

To identify anterior hyaloid proliferation in cases of recurrent vitreous hemorrhage.

MANAGEMENT

- Depends on the cause
- Broad guidelines
- If fresh vitreous hemorrhage, advice bed rest with head end elevated with 2 pillows. Review the patient in 1 week time. If a retinal break is strongly suspected, one can admit the patient for strict bed rest. Bedrest only helps settle the heme down improving the visualization
- If ultrasound is showing an attached retina with no evidence of vitreous traction on the retina one can wait and review the patient again at 1- 2 months time.

Early Surgical Intervention Advocated in

- Bilateral vitreous hemorrhage
- TRD close to/involving macula

- Trauma cases
- One eyed patient
- Vitreous hemorrhage associated with RD
- Nonclearing vitreous hemorrhage > 3 months
- Associated ghost cell glaucoma
- Horseshoe tear visualized on ultrasound
- Posterior pole elevated lesion on ultrasound along with vitreous hemorrhage in elderly age group should commensurate with AMD, confuse with melanoma, breakthrough bleed from subretinal blood
- One need to repeat ultrasound in 10 to 15 days and to look for change in size of mass.

VASCULAR DISEASE—ARTERY AND VEIN OCCLUSION

ACUTE RETINAL ARTERY OCCLUSION

History

- Duration and severity of vision loss
- Predisposing factors, e.g. cardiovascular disease, hypertension, diabetes, coagulation disorders, collagen vascular disease
- Examine old medical records (diagnosis, investigations and treatment elsewhere).

Clinical Examination

- Record vision
- Check for relative afferent pupillary defect (RAPD)
    If you suspect an arterial occlusion try to look through direct ophthalmoscopy.
    - Do a quick fundus evaluation
    - Immediately inform a retina consultant.

Treatment

- Confirmation of diagnosis by retinal specialist
- If the obstruction is within six hours, digital massage should be performed
- Tab Diamox (2 tabs) should be given immediately.
- Anterior chamber paracentesis should be performed
- Carbogen therapy (5% CO_2 and 95% O_2) perform for 10 minutes every 2 hours for 48 hours
- Hyperbaric oxygen therapy (HBOT) can be begun within 2-12 hours of onset
- If the obstruction has occurred more than six hours earlier, the above treatment may not help
- In which case the visual prognosis should be explained and investigations should be ordered.

Investigations

- TLC, DLC, ESR, lipid profile
- Complete cardiac evaluation including Doppler study of carotid, 2 D echography
- To check for hypertension, diabetes, hypercholesterolemia and collagen vascular disorder.

Follow-up

- If massage or paracentesis has been performed then wait for a few hours till the obstruction improves, if not, evaluate him the next day
- Referral to physician if abnormality detected in investigations
- Follow-up every month for first 6 months and then 3 monthly.

CENTRAL RETINAL VEIN OCCLUSION (INCLUDING HEMICENTRAL RETINAL VEIN OCCLUSION)

History

- Duration of loss of vision
- History of pain, redness, congestion
- History of laser treatment elsewhere
- History of diabetes, hypertension and glaucoma
- History of bleeding disorders.

Examination

- Best corrected visual acuity
- Look for RAPD
- Rubeosis iris
- Intraocular pressure
- Gonioscopy to rule out angle neovascularization.

Fundus Examination

- Record severity and extent of retinal hemorrhages
- Venous dilation and tortuosity
- Status of the macula–macular edema, hemorrhages
- Optic disc status–is there any NVD, cupping?

- Is there any glaucomatous cupping in the fellow eye?
- Is there any vitreous hemorrhage?
- Are there any vitreous cells?
- Is there any evidence of perivasculitis?

Investigations

- Fundus Photo–wide angle
- FFA–If the retinal hemorrhages are not severe enough to obscure most of the retinal details
- ERG.

Laboratory Investigations

- Hemoglobin
- TLC, DLC, ESR
- PCV
- Blood smear
- Sickle cell preparation
- Coagulation work-up–bleeding time, clotting time, KCT, prothrombin time, partial thromboplastin time
- If PTT raised or if systemic condition warrants:
  - Antiphospholipid antibody
  - Anticardiolipin antibody IgG, IgM
- Plasma homocysteine by HPCL
- If there is family history of thrombosis or recurrent thrombosis or thrombosis at multiple sites
  - Protein C assay
  - Activated protein C resistance
- Blood sugar estimation.

Treatment

All fresh cases of central retinal vein occlusion (CRVO) have to be followed up on a monthly basis. Follow up continued till there is evidence of resolution of CRVO in the form of development of collaterals, clearing of the retinal hemorrhages, resolution of the macular edema.

At Each Visit Do

- BCVA
- Applanation tonometry
- Slit-lamp evaluation to rule out rubeosis
- Gonioscopy to rule out angle neovascularization
- Fundus evaluation to rule out any neovascularization
- FFA if there is clinical suspicion of neovascularization.

Panretinal Photocoagulation

Done when there is evidence of neovascularization in the eye.

Peripheral Cryo Ablation

- When the neovascularization fails to resolve despite maximum photocoagulation, or a hazy media precludes photocoagulation
- Treatment of glaucoma if indicated
- Treatment of the underlying systemic disorder, if present
- Chorioretinal anastomosis can be considered in selected cases of nonischemic CRVO–RAPD estimation, FFA, ERG mandatory in these cases.

For Macular Edema

- Anti-VEGF agents
- Intravitreal triamcinolone acetonide (IVTA)
- Dexamethasone intravitreal implant.

BRANCH RETINAL VEIN OCCLUSION

History

- Duration of loss of vision
- History of laser treatment elsewhere
- History of diabetes, hypertension and glaucoma
- History of bleeding disorders.

Examination

- Best corrected visual acuity
- Look for RAPD
- Rubeosis of iris
- Intraocular pressure.

Fundus Examination

- Record severity and extent of retinal hemorrhages
- Venous dilatation and tortuosity
- Is there evidence of NVD/NVE
- Status of macula–Macular edema, hemorrhages
- Optic disc status–if there is NVD or cupping
- Is there glaucomatous cupping in the fellow eye?
- Is there vitreous hemorrhage?
- Is there evidence of perivasculitis?

Investigations

- Fundus photo-wide angle
- FFA - If retinal hemorrhages are not severe enough to obscure the retinal details.

Treatment

All fresh cases of branch retinal vein occlusion (BRVO) have to be followed once in 2 months. Follow-up continued till there is evidence of resolution of BRVO in the form of development of collaterals and clearing of retinal hemorrhages, resolution of the macular edema.

Laser

- *Sector panretinal photocoagulation:* Done when there is neovascularization in the eye
- *Grid laser photocoagulation:* Done when there is angiographic evidence of macular edema, persisting for more than 3 months if vision is less than 6/12
- Intravitreal anti-VEGF and IVTA/Dexamethasone implants for the management of macular edema.

DIABETIC RETINOPATHY

HISTORY

- Symptoms (blurring, distortion, difficulty with night vision or reading, floaters)
- Age of onset of diabetes
- Duration of diabetes
- Glucose status (hemoglobin A_{1c})
- Medications
- Medical history (onset of puberty, obesity)
- Renal history
- Systemic hypertension
- Pregnancy status of women under 50 years old
- Serum lipid levels
- Family history
- Social history (alcohol, cigarettes).

EXAMINATION

- Best corrected visual acuity
- Ocular alignment and motility
- Pupil reactivity and function
- Slit lamp examination with high magnification to rule out rubeosis iridis
- *Intraocular pressure:*
  - Gonioscopy when indicated (e.g. neovascularization of the iris or increased intraocular pressure)
- *Fundus evaluation:*
  - Indirect ophthalmoscopy
  - Slit-lamp biomicroscopy of the posterior pole mandatory.

INVESTIGATIONS

- Fundus photograph (7 field fundus photography)
- Fundus fluorescein angiography
- Ultrasound
- Optical coherence tomography (OCT).

Use of Fluorescein Angiography for Diabetic Retinopathy

Situation	Yes	Occasionally	No
Guiding treatment of CSME	•		
Evaluating unexplained visual loss	•		
Determining extent of peripheral capillary nonperfusion		•	
Searching for subtle neovascularization		•	
Screening patient with no or minimal diabetic retinopathy			•

Role of Optical Coherence Tomography

- Detection of macular edema
- Monitoring of macular edema
- Quantification of macular edema (retinal thickness)
- Evaluation of vitreo-macular interface
- ✓ Use of ultrasonography for diabetic retinopathy patients—performed when media opacities preclude exclusion of retinal detachment by indirect ophthalmoscopy.

TREATMENT

- To emphasize the need for strict control of systemic conditions - diabetes, hypertension, nephropathy, hypercholesterolemia, etc.
- To emphasize need for regular follow up
- Laser photocoagulation - Focal grid/Modified Grid for clinically significant macular edema (CSME)
- *Panretinal photocoagulation for proliferative diabetic retinopathy (PDR):*
  - If CSME and PDR coexist, then treat CSME first followed by panretinal photocoagulation 3-4 weeks later
  - If CSME coexists with severe PDR changes, then treat CSME and do 1-2 sitting of panretinal photocoagulation (preferably on the nasal side) followed by further PRP 3-4 weeks later.

Severity of retinopathy	Presence of CSME	Follow-up (months)	Panretinal photocoagulation (Scatter) laser	Fluorescein angiography	Focal and/or grid laser
1. Normal or minimal NPDR	No	12	No	No	No
2. Mild-to-moderate NPDR	No	6-12	No	No	No
	Yes	2-4	No	Usually	Usually
3. Severe NPDR	No	2-4	Sometimes	Rarely	No
	Yes	2-4	Sometimes	Usually	Usually
4. Non-high-risk PDR	No	2-4	Sometimes	Rarely	No
	Yes	2-4	Sometimes	Usually	Usually
5. High-risk PDR	No	2-4	Usually	Rarely	No
	Yes	2-4	Usually	Usually	Usually
6. Inactive/involuted PDR	No	6-12	No	No	Usually
	Yes	2-4	No	Usually	Usually

- Management of diabetic macular edema
  - IVTA/Anti-VEGF agents
  - Focal/Grid laser
  - Combination therapy- Laser + Intravitreal agents
- Vitrectomy
- Low visual aids in burnt out cases
- ✓ In pregnant women, one-eyed patients with other eye lost due to PDR, in patients in whom follow-up cannot be relied upon.

Follow-up

Recommended eye examination schedule for patients with diabetes:

Age of onset of diabetes mellitus (Years)	Recommended time of first exam	Recommended follow-up
0-29	5 years after onset	Yearly
30 and older	At time of diagnosis	Yearly
Prior to pregnancy	Prior to conception or early in the first trimester	No retinopathy to nonsevere NPDR: every 3–12 months Other stages of diabetic retinopathy: every 1-3 months

The follow-up evaluation includes a history and examination.

A follow-up history should include changes in the following:
- Vision
- Medical status
- Glucose control medications and control regimen
- Glucose status
- Other medications
- Ocular history.

A follow-up examination should include the following elements:

- Best corrected visual acuity
- Intraocular pressure
- Slit lamp biomicroscopy with iris examination
- Gonioscopy (if iris neovascularization is suspected or present or if intraocular pressure is increased
- Stereoexamination with biomicroscopy of the posterior pole
- Peripheral retina.

Indications for Vitrectomy

- Vitreous hemorrhage of greater than 3 to 4 months duration–earlier in IDDM cases
- TRD involving/threatening fovea
- Bilateral vitreous hemorrhage
- Presence of combined retinal detachment
- PDR not responding to laser/cryo treatment
- Premacular hemorrhage
- Anterior hyaloid proliferation.

MANAGEMENT OF A CASE OF MACULAR DISORDERS—MACULAR HOLE, EPIRETINAL MEMBRANE AND VITREOMACULAR TRACTION SYNDROME

MACULAR HOLE

History

- History of central scotoma/metamorphopsia
- Duration of visual loss
- History of trauma
- History of episodes of pain, redness in the eyes
- History of wearing glasses
- History of any previous ocular surgery
- Bilaterality of visual complaints.

Examination

- Best corrected visual acuity (BCVA)
- Slit lamp–look for keratic precipitates (KPs), anterior chamber (AC)/vitreous cells, lens clarity
- Intraocular pressure
- *78 D examination:*
  - Stage of macular hole (judge the size, presence or absence of PVD)
  - Any associated SRF cuff
  - Underlying RPE alterations
  - Any associated ERM, operculum
- *I/O examination:*
  - Disc and retinal status
  - Any peripheral retinal degeneration/breaks
  - Any evidence of pars planitis
  - Watzke-Allen test - positive/negative.

Investigations

- Color fundus photography
- *Spectral domain optical coherence tomography (SD-OCT):*
  - Size of hole
  - Whether edge of the hole is raised/flat

- Presence or absence of PVD
- Hole forming factor

Indications for Surgery

- *Idiopathic macular holes:*
  - Stage 2, 3 and 4 macular hole
  - Duration < 6 months
  - Healthy underlying RPE
- *Post-traumatic macular hole:*
  - Duration < 6 months
  - Healthy underlying RPE
  - To wait 2 to 3 months for spontaneous hole closure in pediatric age group.

Surgery not Recommended in

- Large macular holes (> ½ DD)
- Chronic and old macular holes
- Marked underlying pathology, viz. RPE atrophy, choroidal rupture, scarring, etc.

Preoperative Discussion

- Inform patient regarding need for postoperative prone
- Positioning for at least 14 hours a day for 2 weeks
- Possibility of lens changes occurring postoperative
- Avoiding air travel in postoperative period
- Possibility of nonclosure/recurrence of macular hole, RD
- Option of silicone oil in patients who need to undertake immediate air travel or cannot maintain prone position.

EPIRETINAL MEMBRANE

History

- History of metamorphopsia
- Duration of visual loss
- History of trauma
- History of episodes of pain, redness in the eyes

- History of seeing black spots in front of the eyes
- History of undergoing any laser procedure or ocular surgery
- History of having systemic disease like diabetes mellitus.

Examination

- BCVA
- Slit-lamp–look for KPs, AC/Vitreous cells, lens clarity
- AT
- *78 D examination:*
  - Presence or absence of PVD
  - Presence of cellophane maculopathy/epiretinal membrane
  - Presence of ILM folds/CME
  - Underlying RPE-RPE alterations
- *I/O examination:*
  - Disc and retinal status
  - Any peripheral retinal degeneration/breaks
  - Any evidence of pars planitis.

Investigations

Spectral domain optical coherence tomography:
- Presence/absence of epiretinal membrane (ERM)
- Presence or absence of PVD
- Underlying macular changes such as hole, CNV, cystoid changes.

Indications for Surgery

- VA < 6/18, this cut-off would depend on the patients visual requirement
- Presence of mature membrane.

Preoperative Discussion

- Inform patient regarding need for postoperative prone positioning for at least 14 hours a day for 2 weeks, if break occurs and oil or gas has to be injected

- Possibility of lens changes occurring postoperative
- Possibility of recurrence.

VITREOMACULAR TRACTION SYNDROME
History

- History of metamorphopsia/micropsia
- Duration of visual loss
- History of seeing flashes of light.

Examination

- BCVA
- Slit-lamp–look for KPs, AC/Vitreous cells, lens clarity
- Intraocular pressure.

78 D Examination

- Presence or absence of PVD
- Presence of focal or broad attachment of PVD to macula
- Presence of ILM folds/CME
- Underlying RPE-RPE alterations.

I/O Examination

- Disc and retinal status
- Any peripheral retinal degeneration/breaks
- Any evidence of pars planitis.

Investigations

- *Spectral domain optical coherence tomography:*
  - Focal/Broad attachment
  - Whether underlying retina is pulled up and edematous
- *Indications for surgery:*
  - VA < 6/18
  - Presence of broad/multiple vitreoretinal attachment which is unlikely to resolve on it's own
  - Presence of focal vitreoretinal attachment which has persisted for more than 3 months
  - Significant visual disturbance

- *Preoperative discussion:*
  - Goal of surgery is stabilization of vision
  - Inform patient regarding need for postoperative prone positioning for at least 14 hours a day for 2 weeks, if break occurs and oil or gas has to be injected
  - Possibility of lens changes occurring postoperative.

EMERGENCY VITREORETINAL CASES AND MANAGEMENT OF A CASE OF INTRAOCULAR FOREIGN BODY

INTRAOCULAR FOREIGN BODY

In Emergency (Acute presentation)

- Rule out life-threatening systemic injury requiring immediate attention
- Medicolegal consent
- Record vision.

History

- Details of injury–time, mode, circumstances, work setting, suspected foreign body (BD) material, magnetic properties, chances of contamination
- Visual status–prior to and after injury
- *Previous records–treatment received:*
  - Medical and surgical
  - Prophylaxis–antibiotics, tetanus
  - Investigations done—X ray, ultrasonography, CT scan
- Fellow eye status
- Systemic diseases/Drug allergies.

Examination

- Gentle examination–to rule out obvious globe rupture
- Avoid further damage to injured globe. If obvious globe rupture/open wound - patch eye, use rigid shield, avoid all topical medication and contact examinations (AT)
- Document all findings–examination of adnexa, VA, Slit-lamp examination for entry wound, localized corneal edema, (gonioscopy in cases if FB in angle suspected) undilated iris examination, signs of endophthalmitis, pupils for afferent pupillary

defect, lens examination for cataract and embedded foreign body
- Fundus examination with indirect ophthalmoscopy
- Refer to VR emergency (inform duty consultant after OPD hours).

IN VITREORETINAL DEPARTMENT

- Counter check–history and all clinical findings
- Vision especially if noted to be no perception of light or projection of rays inaccurate
- Document all additional findings
- USG–all cases with no view of the fundus, unless open globe.
- Ultrasound biomicroscopy (UBM)–look for FB behind iris and ciliary body region
- CT orbit and brain - Suspected foreign body not localised on USG.
  - Helical CT without contrast
  - Thin slices 0.625–1.25 mm slices
- Foreign body in proximity to ocular coats
- Multiple foreign bodies suspected
- MRI contraindicated in presence of metallic foreign body
- General anesthesia clearance - physician in OPD hours/anesthetist after OPD hours
- To give instructions regarding preoperative fasting if surgery is scheduled for same day.

Treatment

- Admit–all cases requiring wound repair with foreign body removal
- Suspect/frank endophthalmitis
- Tetanus prophylaxis–if not adequately immunized
- IV antibiotics
- Consent for surgery
- Operating surgeon to see patient in the ward prior to surgery.

Immediate Surgery

- Acute presentation requiring wound repair
- Reactive/Vegetative FB
- Suspect/Frank infection
- Prophylactic intravitreal vancomycin + Ceftazidime should be given.

Elective Surgery

- Primary wound repair done elsewhere
- Relatively inert FB
- No suggestive of infection
- Conservative
- Longstanding nonreactive inert encapsulated intraocular foreign body
- Absence of toxicity (Serial ERG, close follow-up).

Emergency Vitreoretinal Cases

- Macula attached RD
- Giant retinal tear
- Postoperative inflammation
- Endophthalmitis
- Patients with IOFB with infection
- One eyed or bilaterally poor vision patients
- Patients with nucleus drop
- Postpenetrating injury
- ROP
- Intraocular cysticercosis
- Intraocular tumors.

ACQUIRED MACULAR DISEASE— CENTRAL SEROUS CHORIORETINOPATHY, AGE-RELATED MACULAR DEGENERATION

CENTRAL SEROUS CHORIORETINOPATHY

History

- Onset and duration of symptoms
- History of blurred vision, metamorphopsia, and color desaturation
- Use of steroids- systemic, ocular injections, topical, or skin ointments, inhalers
- Examine old medical records [diagnosis, investigations-fundus fluorescein angiography (FFA) if done, and treatment]
- *Systemic conditions:* Asthma, skin disease, hypertension, systemic lupus erythematosus (SLE), endocrine disorders, pregnancy, type A personality, status postorgan transplant.

Clinical Examination

- Best corrected visual acuity
- Refraction
- Anterior segment examination and applanation tonometry
- Dilate both eyes-fundus examination with indirect ophthalmoscope and slit-lamp biomicroscopy (78 D)
- Review previous reports and FFA if done elsewhere
- *Note the fundus findings:*
  - *Neurosensory retinal detachment:* Location, extent; presence of shifting fluid, subretinal fibrin, subretinal precipitates
  - *Retinal pigment epithelium (RPE) detachment:* Number, size, RPE atrophic tracts
  - *Rule out secondary conditions:* Choroidal neovascular membranes

- Choroiditis, uveal effusion, Harada's disease, posterior scleritis, optic nerve pit, polypoidal choroidal vasculopathy and choroidal tumor.

Advise Investigations

- Color fundus photograph and fundus fluorescein angiogram. Review FFA and note number and exact site of leaks
- OCT–Optical coherence tomography, scan protocol– macula
- Fundus autofluorescence–where FFA is contra-indicated.

Optional Investigations

- Indocyanine green angiography (ICG)
- Humphrey visual field (HVF): Macular threshold
- Contrast sensitivity functional acuity contrast (FACT)
- Color vision: FM 100 Hue.

Treatment

Observation and Regular Follow-up

- Stop steroids in all forms (if the patient is on high dose, first taper and then stop).
- Call the patient for review after a month and then plan treatment if required.

Indications

- Loss of vision in other eye due to various reasons including central serous retinopathy (CSR)
- Long-standing CSR (more than 3 months)
- If there is a need for early visual recovery (occu-pational)
- If steroids cannot be discontinued because of systemic condition

Options

Argon Green Laser

- For extrafoveal and juxtafoveal leak
- All the leaks must be treated
- *Settings:* Spot size 100-200µ, duration 0.1 second, single pulse
- Power adjusted to get a light white/gray burn.

Photodynamic therapy

- For subfoveal, juxtafoveal leaks
- Low fluence preferred to prevent collateral damage, believed to be effective only in eyes with choroidal hyperfluorescence -ability on ICG.

Prognosis

Depends upon the presenting vision, chronicity and associated structural damage of the fovea.

Follow-up

- The patient is seen after 1 month
- Then at 3, 6, 9 and 12 months
- At every visit a complete examination is done including refraction, IOP measurement, and fundus examination
- OCT
- FFA (if there is persistent neurosensory detachment and if your planning to treat)
- Contrast sensitivity test, fields and FM100 Hue tests are repeated if needed
- Patients in steroid taking group
- If improvement is seen on discontinuing steroids, continue observation.
- If worsening is noted, consider laser treatment
- Patients who are not taking steroids and not treated with laser
- If they do not show improvement in 3 months, consider laser treatment.
- Obliteration of all leaks on repeat FFA indicates successful laser treatment
- Patients with persistent or new leaks may be retreated.

Note

- Preferably use NSAIDs (instead of steroids) in the postoperative period for patients with central serous chorioretinopathy (CSCR) who have to undergo an intraocular surgical procedure.

AGE-RELATED MACULAR DEGENERATION
History

- Duration of visual problems
- Metamorphopsia
- Decreased vision
- Old record of vision in the affected eye
- Previous angiograms, fundus photos
- History of any other eye disease
- History of allergy especially to fluorescein and iodine-related compounds
- Family history of age-related macular degeneration (ARMD)
- Systemic hypertension, smoking
- Past ocular history–any treatments (intravitreal injections, laser)
- Recent history of stroke and myocardial infarction (MI).

Examination

Before Dilatation

- Best corrected visual acuity
- Amsler's grid charting.

After Dilatation

- Indirect ophthalmoscopy (peripheral retinal lesions require prophylactic barrage laser prior to intravitreal injections)
- Slit-lamp biomicroscopy - 78 D.

Specifically Note

- Drusen–hard, soft, confluent
- RPE hyperplasia, RPE rip

- RPE atrophy–geographical and nongeographical
- Choroidal neovascular membrane (CNVM)–Type 1 (sub RPE), Type 2 (subretinal),
- Lipid exudates
- Subretinal fluid
- Retinal edema
- Hemorrhage—subretinal, intraretinal, sub RPE
- Pigment epithelium detachment (PED)—location, serous/turbid/drusenoid/hemorrhagic, notched
- Cystoid macular edema
- Extent of scarring/fibrosis
- Any other pathology that could compromise final visual outcome, e.g. optic atrophy

Investigations

- Fundus photograph–30 degree centered at the fovea
- Fundus fluorescein angiography to define lesion morphology
- *OCT - CNVM:* Look for location, associated features indicating activity such as sub/intraretinal fluid, pigment epithelial detachment, retinal thickening, cystoid macular edema
- Indocyanine green—in occult, polypoidal choroidal vasculopathy, RAP lesions.

Treatment

Dry Age-related Macular Degeneration

- Stop smoking
- Home Amsler's chart
- Glass prescription
- Low visual aids if needed
- To stress importance of a regular retinal evaluation– immediate check-up if any change noted in the Amsler's chart or a routine evaluation every 3 to 6 months
- Earlier check up can be advised if high risk drusens are noted
- Dietary advice
- Explain regarding role of antioxidants

- Vitamin supplements—intermediate drusens, fellow eye disciform scar
- Geographical atrophy.

Wet Age-related Macular Degeneration

Monotherapy: Intravitreal injections of anti-VEGF–ranibizumab (Lucentis), pegaptanib sodium (Macugen), Bevacizumab (Avastin), triamcinolone acetonide.

Indications

- Any type of active CNVM
- Intravitreal injections are given in the operation theater under sterile precautions
- Current dosage regimen - loading dose (3 monthly injections) followed by PRN basis
- Pros and cons of each injection (including off label status if Avastin being used) has to be explained in detail
- Informed consent to be taken
- Follow-up is done every 4-6 weeks.

Combination Therapy

Anti-VEGF/steroids along with PDT.

Indications

- Small classic subfoveal or juxtafoveal CNVM with good vision
- Intravitreal injection is given 2 days after the PDT in the operation theater with dim illumination. Avoid examination with indirect ophthalmoscope/SLE for first one week.

Below Mentioned Treatments can also be Considered

- *Argon laser photocoagulation:* Extrafoveal membranes.
- *Transpupillary thermotherapy:*
  - Subfoveal membranes
  - Juxtafoveal membranes.

Criteria for Retreatment

- Increase in size of the CNVM
- Increase in central retinal thickness
- Persistence of SRF
- Presence of new subretinal hemorrhage
- Decrease in vision by 5 letters in ETDRS chart.

Photodynamic Therapy

- All treatment to be preferably done within 24 to 36 hours of the last angiogram
- To inform patients regarding the possibility of drop in vision following treatment
- To inform patients regarding the occurrence of a scotoma in the central visual field following treatment
- To explain to the patient regarding the chances of recurrence and the possible need for retreatments
- To stress the importance of a re-evaluation after 12 weeks of laser therapy
- To explain risk of photosensitivity on exposure to bright light
- An information booklet is provided to the patient which explains Do's and Don'ts to the patient
- ✓ Currently reduced/half fluence PDT preferred in selective cases (Light intensity-300 mw/cm^2, Energy 25 mJ/cm^2, 83 seconds).

Lesion type (Subfoveal/juxtafoveal)	Combination therapy	Anti-VEGF monotherapy
Classic CNVM		
Small with good VA	✓	✓
Large	-	✓
Occult CNVM		✓
PCV	✓	

INTRAVITREAL INJECTIONS

ANTIBIOTICS/STEROIDS

Indications

Endophthalmitis-Exogenous/Endogenous

Dilution Guidelines

- *Dilute each drug separately*: Balanced salt solution/ Normal saline/Sterile water for injection (preferred) can be used for dilution.
  Note: avoid balanced salt solution, normal saline for diluting amphotericin B in view of precipitation
- Follow the protocol (given below)
- Prepare immediately prior to use, containing the dose to be administered in 0.1 ml final volume
- The volume prepared should be at least 1 cc to reduce dilution error
- Draw up to 0.1 ml of final dilution plus an over fill of 0.05 ml in each syringe to allow placement of the needle (30 G) without loss of dose
- Only 0.1 ml volume is injected
- Preferably use separate syringes for injection of drugs, if injecting more than one drug.

Routes of Administration

- *Trans Limbal:* In aphakic eye
- *Trans pars plana:* In phakic/pseudophakic or aphakic eye with intact posterior capsule.

Method of Administration

- OPD procedure (In operation room, intraoperatively immediately after vitrectomy)
- Topical anesthesia
- Clean the eyelids and periorbital area with iodine preparation
- Enter the vitreous cavity with 30 G needle (mounted on tuberculin syringe, containing desired

drug), either through limbus or pars plana in aphakic eyes and through pars plana in phakic eyes (usually in inferotemporal quadrant)
- Reach mid vitreous cavity
- Inject the drug in vitreous cavity drop-by-drop with bevel of the needle facing up
- Combined drug therapy—ideally inject all the drugs separately.
  Note: Avoid combining any other drug with vancomycin.
- Hold the cotton tipped applicator at injection site for few seconds to prevent the leakage
- Check IOP, if IOP is high, AC paracentesis can be performed
- Apply the patch for 2 hours (after instillation of antibiotic eyedrops).

Drugs	Intravitreal dosage (mg) (bolus)	Intravitreal infusion (µl/min)
Aminoglycosides		
Amikacin	0.1–0.2	10
Gentamycin	0.1	8
Netilmicin	0.25	4
Tobramycin	0.4	10
Antifungals		
Amphotericin B	5–10 µg (0.005–0.01 mg)	10-75
Miconazole	0.025	
Fluconazole	0.1	0.005
Voriconazole	0.1	
Cephalosporins		
Cefazolin	2.25	
Cefotaxime	2	
Ceftazidime	2.25	
Cephaloridine	0.25	
Miscellaneous		
Chloramphenicol	2	10
Clindamycin	1	9
Erythromycin	0.5	
Lincomycin	1.5	10

Contd...

Contd...

Drugs	Intravitreal dosage (mg) (bolus)	Intravitreal infusion (µl/min)
Vancomycin	1	20
Penicillins		
Ampicillin	5	
Carbenicillin (Biopence)	0.5–2.0	
Methicillin	2	20
Oxacillin	0.5	10
Penicillin G	200 units	80 units/ml
Steroids		
Dexamethasone	0.4	16–64

Protocol for Dilution

- Gentamycin
- *Required dose:* 80 mcg (0.08 mg)
- 40 mg/ml vial
- Withthdraw 0. 2 ml (8.0 mg) of gentamycin from the vial
- Add 0.8 ml water for injection to make it 1 ml–(1)
- Take 0.1 cc (0.8 mg) of the solution (1) and add water/dexamethasone for injection to make it 1 ml –(2)
- Inject 0.1 ml of the solution (2)
- Repeat injections: (Intravitreal)
- *72-96 hours:* Nonvitrectomized eye
- *12-35 hours:* Vitrectomized eye.

AMIKACIN

- *Required intravitreal dose:* 100-125 mcg
- 250 mg/2 ml vial (i.e. 125 mg/ml)
- Take 0.1 ml (12.5 mg) from the vial
- Add 0.9 cc of water for injection to make it 1 cc–(1)
- Take 0.1 cc (1.25 mg) of solution (1) and make it up to 1 cc with water/dexamethasone for injection– (2)
- Inject 0.1 cc of solution (2) (0.125 mg)
- Repeat injections
- 24 to 48 hours.

CEFAZOLIN

- *Recommended intravitreal dose:* 2.25 mg
- 500 mg vial
- Add 2 ml of sterile water/saline for injection to the vial-(1) (Total concentration will be 225 mg/ml)
- Withdraw 0.1 ml (22.5 mg) of this solution (1) and add 0.9 ml of sterile water/saline/dexamethasone for injection to make it 1 ml-(2)
- Inject 0.1 ml of solution (2)
- Repeat injections
- *48 to 96 hours:* Nonvitrectomized eye
- *7 hours:* Vitrectomized eye.

CEFTAZIDIME

- *Recommended intravitreal dose:* 2.25 mg
- 1 gram vial
- Add 4.0 ml distilled water/BSS to the vial – (1)
- Take 0.1 ml of solution (1) and add 0.9 ml of distilled water/BSS/dexamethasone to make it 1 ml – (2)
- Inject 0.1 ml of solution (2)
- Repeat injections
- *72 hours:* Nonvitrectomized eye
- *16 hours:* Vitrectomized eye.

VANCOMYCIN

- *Required intravitreal dose:* 1 mg
- 500 mg vial
- Add 5 ml of water for injection (100 mg/ml) to the vial-(1)
- Withdraw 0.1 ml (10 mg) of this solution (1) and add 0.9 ml of water for injection to make it 1 ml – (2)
- Inject 0.1 ml of this solution (2)
- Repeat injections
- *72 hours:* > Nonvitrectomized eye
- *30 hours:* > Vitrectomized eye.

CIPROFLOXACIN

- Available 200 mg/100 ml
- *Required intravitreal dose:* 100 mcg
- Take 0.05 ml from the vial and inject
- Repeat injections depending on clinical course.

AMPHOTERICIN B

- *Recommended intravitreal dose:* 5 mcg
- 50 mg vial
- 1 Add 10 ml distilled water to the vial (5 mg/ml) – (1)
- Take 0.1 ml (500 mcg) of solution (1) and add 0.9 ml distilled water to make it 1 ml – (2)
- Take 0.1 ml (50 mcg) of solution (2) and add distilled water to make l ml – (3)
- Inject 0.1 ml of solution (3)
- Repeat injection
- *11 days:* > Nonvitrectomized eye
- *3-4 days:* > Vitrectomized eye.

VORICONAZOLE

- *Recommended intravitreal dose:* 100 mcg
- 200 mg vial
- Add 19 ml distilled water to the vial (10 mg/ml)-(1)
- Take 0.1 ml (1 mg) of the solution (1) and add 0.9 ml distilled water to make it 1 mg/1 ml-(2)
- Take 0.1 ml (100 mcg) of solution (2) and inject into the vitreous cavity
- Repeat injection
- 48 hours.

DEXAMETHASONE

- *Required intravitreal dose:* 0.4 mg
- Withdraw 0.1 ml from the vial and inject
- Can be administered along with antibiotics. The final dilution of antibiotics can be done with dexamethasone.

MISCELLANEOUS INTRAVITREAL AGENTS
Triamcinolone Acetonide (4 mg/0.1 ml)
Indication

- Diabetic macular edema
- Macular edema due to vascular occlusions
- CME in chronic uveitis.

Anti-VEGF Agents

- Ranibizumab (Lucentis) 0.50 mg in 0.05 ml (pre-filled syringe)
- Bevacizumab (Avastin) 1.25 mg in 0.05 ml
- Pegabtanib (Macugen) 0.34 mg in 0.09 ml (pre-filled syringe)

Indication

- CNVM- AMD/Non AMD
- Prior to diabetic vitrectomy
- Diabetic macular edema
- Macular edema due to vascular occlusions.

Administration Technique

- Prescribe topical broad-spectrum antibiotic eyedrops for 3 days prophylactically (e.g. ciprofloxacin 6 times a day).
- The injection should preferably be injected in the sterile/semisterile environment, with pupillary dilatation.
- *For triamcinolone acetonide:* One can load more than 0.1 ml drug with 26 G needle in a tuberculin syringe, replace with 30 G needle, expel the excess leaving 0.1 ml drug without any air bubble.
- Only 0.1 ml of the drug should be injected.
- *For anti-VEGF:* Load more than 0.05 ml of the drug in a tuberculin syringe, replace with 30 G needle, then 0.05 ml of the drug should be injected.
- Instill one drop of proparacaine into the eye, followed by one drop of betadine eyedrops.

- Clean the eyelids and surrounding area with 5 percent betadine solution.
- Drape the eye with eye hole sheet.
- Apply an appropriate sized eye speculum.
- Request the patient to look straight into the light of the microscope.
- Use your right hand for the right eye of the patient and your left hand for the left eye.
- Hold a cotton tipped applicator/cotton bud soaked in topical lignocaine 4 percent solution, in the other hand and apply it on the conjunctiva in the infero-temporal quadrant for 30 seconds.
- Using the cotton bud move the conjunctiva nasally so that after injection the scleral and the conjunctival openings do not overlap.
- Explain the patient that you are ready to inject and it may be slightly painful, he/she should not move the eye.
- For phakic patients the injection should be given 3.5 mm from the limbus.
- For aphakic and pseudophakic patients should be given 3.0 mm the limbus.
- The direction the needle should be towards the optic nerve head.
- Slowly pierce the sclera, a give way feel shall be experienced once the needle is in the vitreous cavity.
- Visualize the needle tip through the pupil, and inject the drug with the bevel facing towards you.
- Remove the needle gently and cover the injection site with a cotton bud for few seconds.
- Check ocular tension digitally and perform paracentesis if IOP is raised.
- Instill another drop of betadine eyedrops and patch the eye for 2 hours.
- Prescribe topical antibiotic for 3 to 5 days.

RETINOBLASTOMA

HISTORY

Duration of white reflex/squint/change in color of the eye/swelling.

Details of Previous Treatment Received

- Number of chemotherapy cycles (number of drugs, doses, cycles), total radiation done, local consolidation and enucleation
- Family history–siblings of the child/parents/other family members
- History of parental sibling fundus evaluation
- History of bony swellings, loss of weight, vomiting, irritability
- Birth history for differential diagnosis.

Clinical Examinations in the Outpatient Department

- Fix and follow behavior
- Anterior segment examination with 20 D and I/O for ectropion uveae, gross neovascularization of the iris (NVI) feeds visible cilias, proptosis as in retrolenticular fibroplasia, persistent hyperplastic primary vitreous (PHPV)
- Dilated fundus examination–quick scanning of both eyes with child restrained by parents.

Signs to be Noted

- Unilateral or bilateral
- Orbital cellulitis like picture (lid edema, chemosis, congestion of conjunctiva)
- Proptosis
- *Anterior segment involvement:* Iris nodules/pseudo-hypopyon, iris heterochromia/cataract/sub-conjunctival nodules/rubeosis. Visible ciliary processes as in retrolenticular fibroplasias

- Fundus evaluation–gross size of the tumor
- Multifocality, bilaterality
- Endophytic/exophytic
- Associated RD
- Vitreous seeds.

No Mass Lesion

- *Look for telangiectasia (Coats):*
  - Subretinal cholesterol crystals
  - Fibrosis behind lens (RLF, ROP, PHPV).

MANAGEMENT

- *Ultrasound A and B scan:* Both eyes - calcification, document size, optic nerve/extrascleral extension
- MRI–to rule outoptic nerve involvement, intra-cranial disease, metastasis
- Examination under general anesthesia for staging the disease and planning the treatment.

Unilateral Disease

Usually enucleation (after second opinion and signed informed consent)

- *Conservative management (as in bilateral disease) in:*
  - Eyes with vision
  - Tumors away from disc and macula.

Bilateral Disease

- *Conservative treatment:* Near symmetrical involvement of both eyes with no risk factors suggesting enucleation (see below)
- Chemoreduction (2-6 cycles) with sequential aggressive local therapy (SALT)
- *Enucleation (unilateral/bilateral disease):* Histo-pathologic examination (HPE) of specimen reviewed- to decide upon chemotherapy/radiation to the orbit.

Indications of Enucleation

- Eyes without visual potential
- Anterior segment involvement
- Glaucoma
- Orbital cellulitis like appearance
- Tumor > 1/2 the eye (worse eye in bilateral disease to be enucleated)
- Rubeosis.

Always with implant - acrylic/OH and conformer- unless suspecting orbital disease/optic nerve involvement.

Sequential Aggressive Local Therapy—in the Absence of Vitreous Involvement

- Transpupillary thermotherapy - posterior tumors < 3.5 mm.
- Laser photocoagulation - 2 mm thick/3 mm wide .
- Transconjunctival cryopexy - 3 mm thick/4-5 mm wide - peripheral tumors.
- Brachytherapy.

External Beam Radiation

- Response to chemotherapy inadequate
- Involvement of surgical margin of optic nerve
- Orbital recurrence/Metastasis
- Try to avoid in children less than 1 year of age.

Review

- Six weeks if enucleated
- After completion of treatment in chemoreduction
- 6-8 weeks after SALT
- Two months after external beam radiation therapy (EBRT).

Metastatic Work-up

- Proptosis/clinical suspicion of metastasis/optic nerve involvement
- Bone marrow, CSF examination, CT scan (if not already done), bone scan.

Parental/Sibling Evaluation

In all patients with family history/unilateral multifocal disease/bilateral disease [Note down medical record documentation (MRD) numbers in file].

Follow-up

- At least for 5 years of a child with unilateral disease
- Lifelong in familial/genetically transmitted disease.

Genetic Analysis

- In all familial cases
- In children with genetically transmitted disease
- Genetic counseling for familial disease.

CHOROIDAL MELANOMA

Demographics

- The overall mean incidence of uveal melanoma was 4.3 per million
- Higher rate in males (4.9 per million) than in females (3.7 per million)
- Mean age at presentation in the Asian Indian population was found to be 46.1 (range 13-75) years
- Around 150 times more common in whites than in blacks. Less common in Asians
- Usually sporadic rarely inherited
- *Phenotypic associations*: Oculo-dermal melano-cytosis, familial atypical mole and melanoma syndrome, neurofibromatosis type 1 and Li-Fraumeni syndrome.

Clinical Features

- Dome shaped—small and medium-sized tumors are contained by an intact Bruch's membrane. Thickness equal to about half their diameter
- Mushroom or a collar-button shape if Bruch's membrane ruptures at apex.

Tumor Size

Tumor size classifications according to boundary lines are as follows:

- *Small:* Range from 1 mm to 3 mm in apical height and have a basal diameter of at least 5 mm.
- *Medium:* Range from 2 mm to 3 mm up to 10 mm in apical height and have a basal diameter of less than 16 mm.
- *Large:* Greater than 10 mm in apical height or have a basal diameter of at least 16 mm.
- *Diffuse:* Horizontal, flat growth pattern, with the thickness of the tumor measuring approximately 20 percent or less than the greatest basal dimension; this uncommon variant of uveal melanoma seems to have a poorer prognosis.

Differential Diagnosis

Choroidal Neoplasms

- Choroidal nevus
- Choroidal metastasis
- Choroidal hemangioma
- Choroidal leiomyoma.

Hemorrhagic Processes

- Extramacular disciform lesion
- Ruptured arteriolar macroaneurysm.

Retinal Pigment Epithelial Processes

Retinal pigment epithelial hyperplasia.

Inflammatory Processes

Posterior scleritis.

Miscellaneous

- Hemorrhagic retinal detachment
- Intraocular foreign body granuloma.

Optimal Therapeutic Modality

There is still an ongoing debate concerning the optimal therapeutic modality for conserving an eye with uveal melanoma. The options currently available are:
- Enucleation
- Transpupillary thermotherapy
- Episcleral plaque radiotherapy
- Proton beam radiotherapy
- Stereotactic radiotherapy
- Photocoagulation
- Photodynamic therapy with verteporfin
- Cryotherapy
- *Tumor resection:* Trans-scleral resection, endoresection, enucleation
- Ancillary treatments.

Enucleation: It is still the commonest treatment available for choroidal melanoma in our country.

Transpupillary Thermotherapy

- Focused on the target area more precisely than the ionizing radiation
- High rate of late recurrences
- *Sole therapy:* reserved for small tumors less than 3 mm thick
- *Transpupillary thermotherapy (TTT) combined with plaque radiotherapy (sandwich therapy):* TTT destroys the superficial part and radiotherapy treats the deeper portions.

Contraindications

- Media opacities that obscure the retinal image
- Insufficient dilatation of the pupil
- Peripherally located tumors.

Brachytherapy

- The radionuclides used include cobalt-60, ruthenium-106, iodine- 125, palladium-103, gold - 198, iridium-192 and strontium-90

- Accurate estimate of the largest basal diameter is important
- Most centers deliver an apex dose of 80-100 Gy.

Complications

- Cataract
- Optic neuropathy
- Radiation retinopathy
- Neovascular glaucoma
- Scleral melting.

Proton Beam Radiotherapy (Not Available in the Country)

- External beam radiation (EBRT) is usually preferred if tumors are large and/or located near the optic nerve or macula
- If patients are free of metastases, other primary malignancies, and there are no contraindications for surgery, all melanomas, regardless of size or location, are treated with proton therapy.

Contraindications

- Very large melanomas occupying > 30 percent of the ocular volume
- Large extrascleral extensions
- Extensive neovascularization in a painful eye.

Complications

- Rubeosis iridis and neovascular glaucoma
- Retinal detachment
- Radiation retinopathy and papillopathy.

Stereotactic Radiotherapy (Not Available in the Country)

- *Two techniques:* Stereotactic radiosurgery, and fractionated stereotactic radiotherapy
- Radiosurgery is delivered using the Leksell Gamma Knife (LGK)

- Both forms are useful for tumors that are unsuitable for brachytherapy, either because of posterior location or large size.

Contraindication: If the patient does not accept the increased chances of retinal detachment and neovascular glaucoma.

Surgical Resection

Trans-scleral Choroidectomy

- Highly motivated patients with tumor unsuitable for radiotherapy
- Secondary local tumor resection can be useful as a salvage procedure after radiotherapy.

Contraindications

- Any systemic disease that precludes profound hypotensive anesthesia
- Basal tumor diameter greater than 16 mm
- Retinal perforation
- Optic disc involvement
- Invasion of more than three clock hours of the ciliary body or angle.

Extraocular extension is not a contraindication if the tumor is otherwise resectable or treatable with adjunctive radiotherapy.

Follow-up

Patients are advised to have six monthly liver function tests and a yearly chest X-ray, lifelong.

ACUTE POSTOPERATIVE ENDOPHTHALMITIS

HISTORY

- Type of surgery done–ECCE/PKE/IOL/Trabeculectomy/ICCE/Vitrectomy
- *Symptoms:* Pain, DOV, redness
- *Onset of symptoms:* How many days postoperative?
- *History of treatment received elsewhere:* Intravitreal injections/vitrectomy surgery/IOL removal
- Periocular/Systemic focus of infection.

EXAMINATION

- Visual acuity
- Slit lamp–lid edema, conjunctival congestion, chemosis
- Corneal status, corneal edema/epithelial defect, section infiltration, wound leak/bleb
- Suture track, keratic precipitates, hypopyon, fibrin, IOL status
- IOP–By applanation tonometry (if possible) or Finger tension
- Indirect ophthalmoscopy–document visibility of fundus (till 1st/2nd/3rd order vessels).

MANAGEMENT

- Admit patient
- Ultrasound examination if no view of fundus
- Anterior chamber (AC) tap/preferably vitreous tap- for microbiological study.
- Clean periocular region with iodine preparation solution
- Topical anesthetic drops
- Topical povidone iodine drops and wait for 5 minutes
- Separate lids with wire speculum
- Enter the anterior chamber close to the limbus with a 30 G needle mounted on a 1 cc tuberculin syringe

- Aspirate the AC content (aqueous/exudates/hypopyon)–avoid collapse of AC. If a fibrin membrane is occluding the pupil, peel the membrane with the needle
- Topical antibiotic drops
- Eye patched for 1 hour or till intravitreal injection whichever is earlier
- Specimen sent to microbiology laboratory at the earliest for gram staining, KOH wet mount, bacterial and fungal culture and sensitivity
- Polymerase chain reaction (PCR) for eubacterial, panfungal and *Propionibacterium acnes* genome (inadequate sample, chronic endophthalmitis, suspected *P. acne*)
- In case laboratory is closed then inoculate the aspirate into:
  - BHIB media
  - Thioglycolate media.

MEDICAL MANAGEMENT

Intravitreal Injection–Depending on the Laboratory Report

- *If bacterial:*
  - *Gram-positive organism:* Ceftazidime (2.25 mg) + Vancomycin (1 mg) + Dexamethasone (400 µgm)
  - *Gram-negative organism:* Amikacin (100-125 µgm) + Vancomycin (1 mg) + Dexamethasone (400 µgm)
- If fungus in smear, then amphotericin B (5 µgm) or Voriconazole 25-50 µgm.

Topical Medication

- Ciprofloxacin 0.3% (every hour)
- Tobramycin 0.3% (every hour)
- Prednisolone acetate 1%/Betamethasone 0.1% (every hour) (avoided in cases of smear positive for fungus)
- Atropine twice daily.

Systemic Medication

- Tab Ciplox 500 mg b.i.d or Inj Claforan 1 gm b.i.d for 5 days
- Inj Gentamycin 60-80 mg IM b.i.d 5 days. To keep a watch on renal function especially in elderly individuals
- Systemic steroids depending on the severity of inflammation (bacterial infection), to be started 24 to 48 hours after culture negativity for fungus
- If fungal infection–Tab Fluconazole 200 - 400 mg/day for 3 - 4 weeks, to have baseline liver function test and to repeat biweekly
- If both bacteria and fungus undetected–empirical trial of antibiotics with close watch
- Admission to the ward, depending on the severity of the condition
- *Follow up:* 4 - 6 hours/12 -24 hours depending on the severity of inflammation.

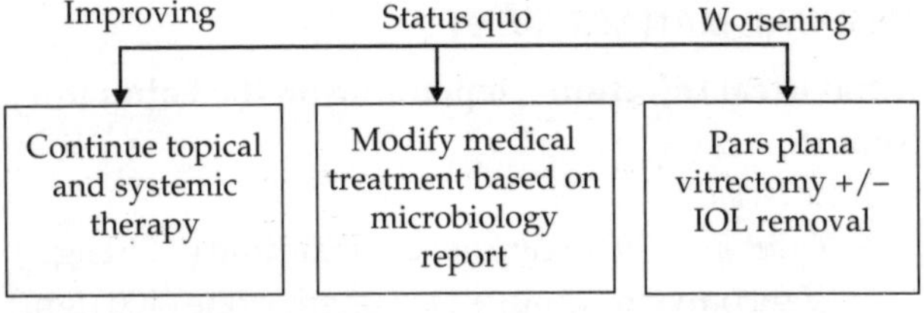

VITRECTOMY

- *Indications:*
  - VA < HMCF
  - Absent fundus glow
  - No response to medical treatment
  - Suspected fungal infection
- *Vitrectomy:*
  - Undiluted vitreous sample is preferred for microbiological analysis 6 mm infusion cannula
  - Send the sample to the laboratory for Gram staining, KOH wet mount, bacterial and fungal culture and sensitivity

- PCR for eubacterial, panfungal and *P. acne* genome
- Give appropriate intravitreal antibiotic at the conclusion of surgery depending upon staining report from the laboratory.

ENDOGENOUS ENDOPHTHALMITIS

History

- Prolonged chronic illness (mainly pulmonary)
- Indwelling catheters
- Recent intravenous infusion
- Blood transfusion
- Immunocompromised patient (Cancer/DM/post-abdominal surgery)
- Known HIV + ve
- Drug abuse
- Prolonged steroid/antibiotic therapy
- Organ transplant (Heart/lung/liver/kidney)
- Systemic focus of infection
- History of cardiac disorder, e.g. bacterial endocarditis
- Chronic renal failure/endoscopic procedures/pelvic inflammatory disease.

Clinical Features

- Variable (ranging from mild vitritis to panophthalmitis)
- Bilateral in 25 percent cases
- Mild-to-severe anterior uveitis with/without hypopyon
- Focal anterior/posterior segment abscess with overlying variable vitritis
- Snow ball vitreous opacities
- Well circumscribed creamy retinal infiltrates
- Intraretinal hemorrhage
- Subretinal abscess
- Papillitis.

Investigations

- Complete physical examination (with special attention to heart, skin and extremities) for systemic focus of infection
- Complete blood count, basic coagulation profile
- Blood culture
- Urine culture
- Wound culture, if present
- CSF culture, in cases with meningitis/encephalitis
- HIV screening, if patient is not a known HIV positive case
- Other ancillary investigations (e.g. CT scan, MRI, Echo, etc.) depending on general examination findings
- Anterior chamber tap for smear/culture
- Vitreous tap/biopsy
- Fine needle aspiration biopsy (FNAB) for subretinal abscess.

Treatment

- Admit patient
- Treat the eye like any other endophthalmitis case
- Nonocular culture sensitivity data will guide initial therapy
- Specific therapy depending on aqueous/vitreous culture and antibiogram report
- Systemic antibiotics (preferably IV)
- Intravitreal antibiotics/steroids
- Topical antibiotics/steroids
- Therapeutic and diagnostic vitrectomy, if necessary
- Systemic antifungals–only if systemic focus of fungal infection is present.

Intravitreal Injections

Please refer to chapters on intravitreal injections for dosages and preparations indication.

Dilution of Intravitreal Drugs

S. No.	Name of the drug	Dilute with	Method of dilution	Steps of dilution in 1 ml syringe
1.	Amphotericin B (50 mg) Intravitreal dose 5 mcg	10 ml water for injection	Double dilution	1. Take 0.1 ml of Ampo 2. Dilute with 0.9 ml of water 3. Mix well 4. Discard 0.9 ml 5. Again take 0.9 ml of water 6. Mix well 7. Discard 0.9 ml 8. Use 0.1 ml for injection
2.	Amikacin 250 mg Intravitreal dose 250 mcg	-	Double dilution If Decadron—second dilution with Decadron	1 to 4 same as above If Decadron 5 Take 0.9 ml of Decadron instead of water Steps 6–8 same as above
3.	Vancomycin (500 mg) Intravitreal dosage 1 mg	5 ml	Single dilution	Steps 1–4 Next step 8

Contd...

Contd...

S. No.	Name of the drug	Dilute with	Method of dilution	Steps of dilution in 1 ml syringe
4.	Ceftazidime 1 gm Intravitreal dose 2.5 mg	4 ml	Single dilution If Decadron, directly dilute with Decadron	Same as vancomycin If Decadron, use Decadron instead of water in steps 1-4
5.	Voriconazole (200 mg) Intravitreal dosage 50 mcg	19 ml	One and half dilution	Steps 1-3 same 4. Discard 0.5 ml 5. Take 0.5 ml of water 6. Mix well 7. Discard 0.9 ml 8. Use remaining 0.1 ml for injection
6.	Gentamycin (80 mg) Intravitreal dosage 80 mcg		Double dilution	1. Take 0.2 ml in 1 cc syringe 2. Dilute with 0.8 cc of water and mix 3. Discard 0.9 cc 4. Dilute with 0.9 cc of water and mix 5. Discard 0.9 cc 6. Inject 0.1 cc
7.	Ciplox (200 mcg/0.1 ml)		No dilution	Take 0.5 ml and inject

OUTPATIENT DEPARTMENT PROCEDURES—ULTRASOUND A AND B SCAN, LASERS AND CRYOTHERAPY

DIAGNOSTIC ULTRASOUND A-SCAN

Indications

Microphthalmos

Clinically some eyes with small corneas are suspected of being microphthalmic when actually the length is normal or increased.

Nanophthalmos

- To diagnose nanophthalmos
- In such cases axial length, lens thickness, choroidal thickness, scleral thickness (B-scan), also should be measured.

Axial Myopia

- To differentiate between axial and lenticular myopia
- In such cases B-scan is helpful in picking up posterior staphylomas
- Vector A-scan with B-scan (Dual A + B mode)
- All the cases of mass lesions A-scan mode to be used with the B-scan
- All cases of IOFBs A-scan mode to be used with B-scan.

B-scan Ultrasound

Indications

Opaque Ocular Media

a. *Anterior segment:*
  - Corneal opacification
  - Hyphema, hypopyon
  - Miosis
  - Pupillary membrane

- Cataract
- Posterior capsular opacification.

b. *Posterior segment:*
- Vitreous hemorrhage
- Endophthalmitis.

Clear Ocular Media

a. *Anterior segment:*
- Iris lesion
- Ciliary body lesions

b. *Posterior segment:*
- Intraocular tumors
- Choroidal detachment (serous versus hemorrhagic)
- Retinal detachment (rhegmatogenous versus exudative)
- Optic disc abnormalities
- Suspected Vogt-Koyanagi-Harada (VKH), posterior scleritis.

c. Intraocular foreign bodies.

Technique

- The patient's name, MRD no., the eye, which is to be examined, is entered on the screen and in patient's record register provided
- Before examination, the notes of the consultant who has asked for the ultrasound should be checked for any specific ultrasound findings required by him
- The patient lies in supine position
- The echographer positions himself on the right side of the patient
- The patient's head and instruments to be used are situated close together, so that the probe position and the screen may be viewed simultaneously
- The patient is asked to close his eyelids and a sterile nonantigenic gel is applied over the closed lids as a coupling medium to ensure sufficient sound penetration
- The ultrasound probe is then placed vertically in contact with the gel for examination.

Ultrasound Probe Orientations (For Ocular Ultrasound)

The probe has a vertical line marker on its shaft; the direction in which the marker is oriented appears topmost on the viewing screen.

Axial Scan

It is performed with the patient fixating in the primary gaze and with the probe face centered on the cornea; thereby displaying the lens and optic nerve in the center of the echogram. It is useful for evaluating posterior lesions. Horizontal axial scan is performed with the marker directed towards the patient's nose for the right eye and away from the nose for the left eye.

Transverse and Longitudinal Scans

- They are performed with the probe lying peripheral to the cornea and with the patient's gaze directed away from the probe, towards the meridian being examined.
- In transverse scan, the probe is positioned such that the axis of the marker lies tangential to the limbus. This orientation is appropriate for showing the lateral (circumferential) extent of the lesion.
- In longitudinal scan, the probe is positioned such that the axis of the marker lies perpendicular to the limbus. This orientation is ideal to show the anteroposterior extent of the lesion.
- After having examined the eye a printout which is most representative of the pathology is taken and attached to the patient's file; the examiner also notes his findings and impression of the lesion, especially dynamic features.

    In postoperative patients and open globe injuries, the probe is cleaned with Bacillocid solution before examination and the examination should be performed gently.
- In infected cases, the probe should be cleaned as mentioned above, both before and after use.

Interpretation

In Trauma Cases

The various aspects to be examined are:

- *Lens:* Location, presence or absence, intralenticular foreign body, subluxation (which direction), dislocation (which location, whether mobile or fixed), if pseudophakic–whether IOL is in place or dislocated, status of the posterior capsule.
- *Vitreous:* Vitreous incarceration, PVD (partial, complete).
- *Retina:* Detachment (whether rhegmatogenous, tractional or combined), giant retinal tear, retinal incarceration.
- *Intraocular foreign body:* Number, size, location (anterior, mid or posterior vitreous cavity and which clock hour), mobile/immobile.
- *Choroid:* Thickening, detachment (extent, nature— serous, hemorrhagic), if hemorrhagic detachment whether organized or liquefied
- *Ocular coats:* Intact, defect (location, incarceration of structures), IOFB in ocular coats.
- *Optic nerve:* Normal, irregular, thickened, FB in the optic nerve
- *Orbit:* Hematoma, FB.

In Vitreous Hemorrhage

- *Echoes:* Type of reflectivity, amount, distribution– whether intragel or subhyaloid, if subhyaloid– whether mobile or fixed.
- *Posterior vitreous detachment:* Present/absent, if present-complete/incomplete, if incomplete-focal/ broad attachment, location of attachment, associated retinal breaks with attachment of vitreous vitreoschisis (location).
- *Retinal detachment:* Present/absent, if present— rhegmatogenous, tractional, combined, if exudative- presence/absence of mass, associated choroidal thickening, shifting fluid, extent of RD, PVR, retinal breaks, giant retinal tear, retinoschisis.

- *Choroidal detachment:* Serous/hemorrhagic, if hemorrhagic-liquefied/organized, extent of choroidal detachment
- *Mass lesion in posterior segment:* ARMD/Intraocular tumor.

In Endophthalmitis

- *Intraocular lens:* Present/absent
- *Intragel echoes:* Nature- dot-like/clump-like/membrane like, location, reflectivity, amount
- *Posterior vitreous detachment:* Present/absent
- *Retinal detachment:* Rhegmatogenous/tractional/exudative
- Choroidal thickening (measure thickness), detachment-note extent and amount
- *T-sign:* Present/absent
- Compare axial lengths of the two eyes
- *If post-traumatic:* Look for IOFB
- *If endogenous:* Look for fluffy ball-like opacities suggestive of fungal etiology, cysticercus cyst, tumor mass (Important: probe to be cleaned thoroughly after examination).

Mass Lesion: If Present

- *Number:* Single/multiple
- *Shape:* Mushroom-shaped, cystic, dome-shaped
- Location
- *Measurements:* Anteroposterior, horizontal, vertical
- Extrascleral extension/choroidal excavation
- *Surface:* Reflectivity, whether regular/irregular, dome-shaped/excavated
- Internal reflectivity
- Evidence of calcification within the mass
- *Associated RD:* Shifting fluid
- Optic nerve involvement
- Associated vitreous changes
- T-sign.

Leukocoria

- *Persistent hyperplastic primary vitreous:* High gain required to pick the central strand, axial lengths of the two eyes should be compared
- *Coats' disease:* Exudative RD, characterize subretinal deposits if any (important to make patient sit-up and check again).

Retinoblastoma

- Calcification
- Vitreous seeding
- Optic nerve involvement
- Compare axial lengths of the two eyes
- If there are multiple tumors each is to be characterized separately.

Retinopathy of Prematurity

- Whether funnel type—funnel open or closed
- Location of loops if any
- Characterize intragel and subretinal echoes
- Peripheral granuloma (*Toxocara*)
- *Cysticercus:* look for scolex
- Ciliary body mass with cystic cavities (Diktyoma).

Postoperative Cases

- *Important:* To clean the probe before examination, and to check operative notes as well as verify what the advising consultant wants to know
- Lens status
- *Vitreous cavity:* Clear/echogenic, if echogenic-characterize the echoes
- *PVD:* Present/Absent
- *RD:* Present/Absent
- *Choroidal thickening/detachment:* If detachment-serous/hemorrhagic
- *In case of intraocular gas:* Do ultrasound in erect position
- *In case of intraocular silicon oil:* Do ultrasound in orbit mode

- *Buckle effect:* Present/Absent, extent
- *Residual vitreous:* Location.

Total Cataract/Corneal Opacity Cases

- Shape of the lens
- Position of the lens
- Integrity of posterior capsule
- Lens droppings in vitreous cavity
- Intralenticular FB in trauma cases
- *Dislocated nucleus:* Fixed/mobile
- Rule out causes of leukocoria (see above)
- *If unilateral cataract:* Check for RD/tumor/choroidal thickening/compare axial lengths
- *Macula:* For disciform scar/macular edema
- *PVD:* Senile/Pathological
- Optic nerve head cupping
- *If complicated cataract:* Look for phthisical changes.

Nanophthalmos

- Axial length
- Choroidal thickness
- Scleral thickness
- Choroidal thickening lens thickness (if possible).

ORBITAL ULTRASOUND

Indications

- *Proptosis:* Orbital mass lesions/vascular malformations
- Thyroid related ophthalmopathy
- *Orbital trauma:* Foreign bodies/hematoma/optic nerve injury
- *Orbital inflammatory diseases:* Cellulitis/abscess/idiopathic orbital inflammation/parasitic infestation.

Technique

- Soft tissue evaluation
- Extraocular muscles
- Retrobulbar optic nerve.

Soft Tissue Evaluation

Scan Methods

- *Transocular:* Lesions in mid and posterior orbit
- *Paraocular:* Lesions in lids and anterior orbit.

Technique

- Positioning - supine
- Compare both orbits always
- B-scan technique.

Transocular

Transverse

For lateral extent of lesion:
- Probe placed tangential to limbus in all meridians
- Horizontal transverse scan always has probe marker facing towards the patient's nose. Vertical transverse scan always has probe marker facing superiorly
- Oblique transverse scans always have probe marker facing upwards.

Longitudinal

- For anteroposterior extent of the lesion
- Probe marker towards center of cornea with probe perpendicular to the limbus in desired meridian
- Axial
- Probe placed over cornea with patient fixating in primary gaze.

Paraocular

- Horizontal
- Vertical
- Oblique
- Paraocular-horizontal and vertical scans

Transverse scans: Probe placed parallel to the orbital wall. Marker directed as for transverse transocular scans. For lateral extent and posterior border of anterior lesions.

Longitudinal scans: Probe placed between the globe and orbital rim, perpendicular to the rim. Marker directed towards globe for inferior meridians, while towards orbital rim for superior meridians.

B-Scan Screening

- Initial transverse transocular scans in four major meridians, in medium-high gain setting.
- Superior orbit is scanned first, with patient looking in up-gaze, beginning form posterior to anterior. This is followed by nasal, inferior and temporal orbit scan in a similar manner.
- Longitudinal transocular scans are used for orbital soft tissue and lacrimal gland.
- Axial scans are used for retrobulbar space.
- Compare both orbits.
- If normal – compare axial length, do Valsalva maneuver to rule out a varix and assess the compressibility of soft tissues.

A-Scan Screening

It can be used in all approaches along with a B-scan.

Special Examination Techniques

Topographic Echography

Topography

- Location, size and shape of lesion.
- Transocular transverse scan for lateral extent, shape and thickness of lesion.
- Longitudinal scan displays the lesion in long section, shape and posterior extension.
- Patient looks towards the lesion and the probe is placed at the opposite limbus, then shifted from limbus to fornix till the center of the lesion is displayed.
- Axial scan displays relation to globe wall, optic nerve, extraocular muscles and orbital bones.

Borders

- *Well outlined:* Smooth, regular contour, rounded shape and a distinct high posterior surface spike.
- *Poorly outlined:* Indistinct irregular contour with lower reflective posterior surface spike.
- Contour changes in globe and bone.
- *Globe indentation/flattening:* Bone excavation/defects/ hyperostosis.

Immersion Technique

Using scleral shell placed directly over the lesion with a coupling solution for small lesions of lids/ conjunctiva and anterior orbit.

Kinetic Echography

- Used for dynamic assessment of motion of or within a lesion.
- *Consistency:* Assessed by compressibility testing. The probe is placed such that the beam is perpendicular to the border of the lesion through its thickest portion. Mild pressure is applied while avoiding change in position of probe/lesion.
- *Vascularity:* With patient fixating on a target, the lesion is displayed in its maximal thickness. The probe is held stationary and intralesional echoes are observed for fast spontaneous flickering movements on A and B scan.
- *Mobility:* Of the lesion or its contents is assessed on a B-scan while patient performs a saccade.

Extraocular Muscles

- *B-scan:* Gross size and contour
- *A-scan:* Precise measurement and internal architecture
- Always compare with other eye at the same settings.

Rectus Muscles
B-scan Technique

- Usually at medium gain settings with patient fixating in the primary gaze/10 degree towards the muscle being examined.
- *Transverse scans:* Cross-section of muscle. Probe is placed near the opposite equator of the globe
- *Longitudinal scans:* Long section of the muscle. Probe placed along the meridian of the muscle at the opposite end with the marker facing towards the center of the cornea.

A-Scan Technique

- At tissue sensitivity settings, attempt to obtain the widest part of the muscle. The beam should be perpendicular to the muscle sheath and will give a steeply rising double peaked spike. Internal reflectivity to be assessed within the anterior 1/3 to 1/2 of the muscle to avoid effects of sound attenuation.
- Measurements to be compared with normal values and those of the other eye.

Oblique Muscles
Superior Oblique

- *Tendon:* B-scan of the superior orbit with probe in horizontal transverse position
- *Muscle:* Oblique transverse B-scan of the superonasal orbit above the medial rectus.
- *Trochlea:* When inflamed can be imaged with a longitudinal B-scan.
- A scan only used if abnormality noted on B-scan.

Inferior Oblique

- *Insertion:* Oblique transverse B-scan of inferotemporal orbit
- *Belly:* Imaged only when thickened. Horizontal transverse B-scan through the inferior orbit is used. Alter-

natively a paraocular B-scan of the inferotemporal orbit is used.

Retrobulbar Optic Nerve
B-Scan Technique

- Used to evaluate general topography, relationship to surrounding structures/lesions and associated abnormalities
- With medium gain setting axial/longitudinal/transverse scans may be used
- Always compare with contralateral nerve

Axial scan: Limited role to detect gross enlargement of the nerve, because of artifactual wedge shaped optic nerve shadow.

Longitudinal scan: Longitudinal scan of the horizontal meridian with the probe placed at the temporal limbus.

Transverse scan: Vertical scan at the temporal limbus can be used to detect gross-thickening of the nerve.

A-Scan Technique

Used to access internal reflectivity and structure of nerve and its sheath.

- At the temporal equator the probe is used to scan the orbit anterior to posterior while the beam is perpendicular to the nerve sheath. The nerve can be traced posteriorly to the extent possible.
- Measurements are made between two inner steeply rising high reflective double peaked sheath spikes.
- Reflectivity is assessed in the anterior half of the nerve to avoid sound attenuation.

Thirty-Degree Test

- A scan technique to differentiate thickening of the nerve with increased subarachnoid fluid.
- If a widened nerve is detected maximum thickness is documented anteriorly and posteriorly in the primary gaze.

- With patient refixating at 30 degree towards the probe the measurements are repeated again after a few minutes. If the measurements reduce compared to the primary gaze, it suggests increased subarachnoid fluid (at least 10% decrease).

SPECIFIC SITUATIONS
Orbital Tumors

- *Location:* Intraconal/extraconal and quadrant.
- *Shape and extent:* Measurements when possible
- *Borders:* Well circumscribed/ill defined
- Internal reflectivity
- *Internal structure:* Solid/cystic
- Sound attenuation
- Vascularity
- Consistency/Compressibility/Change in size with posture
- Ocular indentation/findings
- Extraocular muscles: Normal/involved
- Optic nerve shadow: Normal/widened/irregular/ shifted
- T-sign
- Dilated orbital veins (superior ophthalmic vein)
- Bone.

Note: For FNAB take pictures before and during needle entry.

LASER PROCEDURES IN OUTPATIENT DEPARTMENT

- Indications for photocoagulation:
- Proliferative diabetic retinopathy
- Proliferative vascular retinopathy viz post vasculitis, retinal vein occlusions, ocular ischemic syndrome, familial exudative vitreoretinopathy (FEVR)
- Macular edema due to diabetes, postretinal vein occlusion
- Prophylaxis of retinal detachment

Tumor	Shape	Internal reflectivity	Internal structure	Sound attenuation	Vascularity	Bone
Pseudotumor/Lymphoma	Variable	Low-medium	Regular	Weak	+/−	N
Rhabdomyosarcoma	Variable	Low-medium	Irregular	Moderate	+	N/Defects
Schwannoma	Oval	Low-medium	Regular/Cystic+	Moderate	+	N/Excavated
Neurofibroma	Oval/Irregular	Low-high	Regular/Irregular	Weak/Moderate	+/−	N
Metastasis	Irregular	Variable	Variable	Weak/Moderate	−	N/Defects
Pleomorphic adenoma	Round/Oval	Medium-high	Regular	Moderate	−	N/Excavated
Adenoid cystic carcinoma	Irregular	Medium-high	Irregular	Moderate/Strong	−	Excavated/N
Cavernous hemangioma	Round/Oval	High	Regular	Moderate	−	N
Lymphangioma	Irregular	Low	Irregular	Variable	−	N
Capillary hemangioma	Irregular	High	Irregular	Variable	+	N

- Central serous retinopathy with extrafoveal leaks on FFA
- Extrafoveal polyps in idiopathic polypoidal choroidal vasculopathy (IPCV)
- Certain cases of extrafoveal CNVM
- Ocular tumor related conditions including peripheral retinal angioma, small peripheral retinoblastomas, melanomas
- Certain ocular vascular disorders like macro-aneurysms, retinal telangiectasia, Coats' disease, vasoproliferative tumors
- Laser hyaloidotomy
- Optic nerve head (ONH) pit with macular schisis (recommended diode laser).

Protocol

- Informed consent to be taken
- Pretreatment discussion regarding the aim of the treatment, the procedure and its limitations
- Pretreatment FFA when required, maximum less than 2 weeks old
- Treatment done as per guidelines for specific techniques either through slit-lamp delivery or indirect ophthalmoscope delivery
- Different type of lasers done routinely are focal laser, panretinal photocoagulations, lasers in CSR, laser barrage to horseshoe tears, lattices, laser to tumors
- In general, lenses used for slit lamp delivery are Transequatorial lens, Volk quadraspheric lens, Mainster lens and Area centralis for posterior and macular lasers
- Avoid direct treatment to neovascularizations (NVs), avoid areas of FVP
  Precautions of restricted activity explained in cases of fresh vitreous hemorrhage/signs suggestive of vitreoretinal traction present.

Precautions during lasers are:
- Patient identity, eye rechecked
- Case file reviewed

- Contact lens delivery of laser avoided in early post-operative period
- If in absolute need, lenses are sterilized and used with new gonio lens solution
- Lenses should be washed in between the cases
- Titrate the burns
- Avoid 50 mc burn
- Avoid lens or iris burns
- Avoid macular burn, or burn to any major blood vessel.

Follow-up

- Follow-up generally 2-3 months later
- Earlier if complaining of loss of vision
- Evaluation includes best corrected visual acuity, refraction, fundus examination, color photo, FFA/ICG/OCT/USG if necessary
- Retreatment as per clinical/angiographical evidence.

PHOTODYNAMIC THERAPY

Introduction

Photodynamic therapy (PDT) is a treatment modality in which a nontoxic light-sensitive compound called a photosensitizer is administered and subsequently activated by light exposure to produce photochemical effects in the target area. Selective occlusion of choroidal neovasculature by this therapy causes minimal damage to the neurosensory retina and, therefore, does not induce loss of visual acuity. This benefit allows verteporfin therapy to be used in the large proportion of patients who are not eligible for treatment by laser photocoagulation.

There are two types of PDT:
1. Light dose with standard fluence: 600 mw/cm^2, 50 J/cm^2
2. Light dose with reduced fluence: 300 mw/cm^2, 25 J/cm^2

   There is an increasing trend towards opting for reduced fluence for most of the indications nowadays, due to its lesser tissue damage. Also with the advent of combination therapy, viz. PDT followed by intravitreal anti-VEGF/IVTA after 48 hours, reduced fluence is more in vogue.

Indications

Choroidal Neovascular Membrane

- *Age-related macular degeneration (AMD):* Subfoveal predominantly classic choroidal neovascularization (CNV) (>50% classic CNVM, area not larger than 5400 μm in eyes with a visual acuity of 6/60 or better)
- Classic subfoveal/juxtafoveal CNVM of other etiologies, viz. myopia, parafoveal telangiectasia, angioid streaks, associated with choroidal rupture, Best dystrophy, inflammatory, idiopathic and others.
- Idiopathic polypoidal choroidal vasculopathy (IPCV) with subfoveal/juxtafoveal polyps or atleast some of the polyps being subfoveal/juxtafoveal with less signs of exudation
- Retinal angiomatous proliferation (RAP) with associated CNV
- Recurrent central serous retinopathy with subfoveal and or juxtafoveal leaks
- Vascular tumors, viz. choroidal hemangioma, retinal angioma, vasoproliferative tumors involving the posterior pole especially with associated vision-threatening signs.

Contraindications

- Allergy to porphyrin compounds/verteporfin
- History of porphyria.

Cautions

- History of liver disease
- Pregnancy
- History of intake of other photosensitive medications.

Protocol

- Pretreatment discussion about the aim of the treatment–"Stabilization" of vision (not improvement or maintenance)
- Informed consent to be taken
- Calculations of the dose of the drug based on weight, height, body surface area
- Pretreatment FFA< 1 week old
- Treatment as per guidelines for PDT [intravenous infusion of vertiporphyrin in 5 percent dextrose of 30 ml over 10 minutes; avoiding extravasations of the dye (risk of necrosis)]
- Laser application 5 minutes later
- Patient to remaining indoors and avoid bright sunlight for 48 hours
- Prefer use of long sleeve cloth and dark glasses post-laser.

Follow-up

- Usually after a month especially in case of combination treatment where additional injections are planned
- Earlier follow-up if complaining of loss of vision. Evaluation includes, best corrected visual acuity, refraction, fundus examination, Color Photo, FFA, (ICG/OCT/USG if necessary)
- Retreatment with PDT if persistent leak on FFA (irrespective of visual maintenance/improvement).

TRANSPUPILLARY THERMOTHERAPY

Indications

The current definite indications of TTT are ocular tumors posteriorly located, i.e. choroidal melanoma, circumscribed choroidal hemangioma, and retino-blastoma including the adult onset type. The necessary criterias for treatment are discussed in the respective section.

Protocol

- Pretreatment discussion about the aim of the treatment–"Stabilization" of vision (not improvement or maintenance). Informed consent to be taken.
- Treatment in OPD delivered through slit lamp with large spot adapter of the diode laser.
- Treatment as per guidelines for TTT in Asian eyes (spot size to cover the lesion complex; 1 minute duration burns; Mainster standard lens for CNVM <3 mm; Volk transequatorial lens for CNVM > 3 mm; multiple spots for CNVM larger than that could be treated with the Volk lens; power selection based on available guidelines for Asian eyes; no visible change at the end of the treatment).
- Patient cautioned against activity that may cause subretinal hemorrhage.
- Precautions to be followed for 1 month.

Follow-up

Follow-up 3 months later; earlier if complaining of loss of vision; evaluation includes, best corrected visual acuity, refraction, fundus examination, Color Photo, FFA (ICG/OCT if necessary). Retreatment with TTT if persistent activity noted on clinical/OCT/angiogram.

CRYOTHERAPY

Preferably, transconjunctival cryotherapy is performed after physician's clearance under local anesthesia. The procedure is done in the operation theater under monitoring of vitals.

Indications

- Prophylaxis of retinal detachment, especially in cases with hazy media.
- Anterior retinal cryo when neovascularizaton fails to resolve despite maximum photocoagulation.
- Anterior retinal cryo in nonresolving vitreous hemorrhage of 1 to 2 months of duration due to

proliferative diabetic retinopathy with maximum panretinal photocoagulation done and especially when the hemorrhage is not dense.
- Ocular tumors including peripheral small Retinoblastoma, Coats' disease.

Protocol

- Pretreatment discussion of the aim of the treatment, the procedure and its limitations.
- Informed consent to be taken both for cryo as well as local anesthesia.
- Treatment as per guidelines for specific indications. After local anesthesia, speculum is put and transcleral cryo done. For tumors triple freeze thaw technique is used. ARC can be done in 2 separate sittings, inferior half first and superior half if required after 2 to 3 weeks.
- Antibiotic ointment put at the end of the procedure with a patch for 4 hours if local anesthetic has been given.
- Procedure done on day care basis and the patient is put on systemic analgesics and local steroid drops for 1 to 2 weeks.

Follow-up

- Follow-up 3 weeks to 2 months depending on the indication
- Evaluation includes, best corrected visual acuity, refraction, fundus examination, FFA/OCT/USG if necessary.

8

Ocular Trauma

- Open Globe Injuries
- Chemical Injuries
- Closed Globe Injuries
- Traumatic Optic Neuropathy
- Eyelid and Adnexal Injuries
- Orbital Injuries Including Fractures
- Guidelines for the Emergency Doctors

OPEN GLOBE INJURIES

- Corneal laceration
- Corneoscleral laceration
- Globe rupture
- Intraocular foreign body (IOFB).

An open globe injury is an ophthalmic emergency.

HISTORY

- *Nature of the injury:*
  - Accidental
  - Self-inflicted
  - Assault.
- *Cause of the injury:*
  - Industrial accidents
  - Domestic accidents
  - Others.
- *In case of foreign body:*
  - Composition
  - Dimension of the foreign body.
- *Treatment history:*
  - Medical—use of any medications, antibiotics (systemic), tetanus prophylaxis, antibiotics (topical).
  - Surgical procedure including primary wound repair.

EXAMINATION

- Reassure the patient—make them comfortable and handle them gently.
- Check visual acuity first.
- Use sterile disposable gloves for examination.
- Clean ooze/discharge/external contamination carefully with sterile gauze.
- Lids to be separated very gently for slit-lamp examination.

- For pediatric cases—minimal manipulation/torch light examinations. Rest of the details to be evaluated under general anesthesia (GA).
- Look for any associated facial asymmetry/lid and adnexal trauma/enophthalmos/proptosis.
- Look for any evidence of infections—lid edema, purulent discharge, etc.
- Examine the pupils and check for relative afferent pupillary defect (RAPD) in all cases.
- Inform trauma/duty consultant for help if required.
- Check for extraocular movement—in open globe state, do not check for ocular motility, since this can lead to raised intraocular pressure and extrusion of ocular contents.

Corneal/Corneoscleral Lacerations

- Always look for the posterior extent of the laceration, if possible.
- Determine whether the laceration is full thickness or partial thickness. If in doubt look for anterior chamber depth/perform forced Siedel's test.
- Measure the dimensions of the laceration and represent the same with a diagram.
- Record other anterior segment details like, anterior chamber reaction, blood in anterior chamber, status of the lens, uveal prolapse, vitreous prolapse, etc.
- Do not perform intraocular pressure measurement in open globes.
- Defer fundus examination in open globes (in self-sealed injuries fundus examination can be done with minimal manipulation and no scleral indentation).
- USG can be done in self-sealed lacerations. Defer in open globes.

Globe Ruptures

- Suspect globe rupture in cases with dense subconjunctival hemorrhage, subconjunctival pigment and soft eye.

- Examination is the same as in corneal laceration except that the patient may be advised CT scan to rule out foreign body and associated orbital injuries where appropriate.

Intraocular Foreign Bodies

- History regarding the dimension of the foreign body, composition (magnetic or non-magnetic).
- Patients with penetrating trauma with the history of injury with flying objects should be advised CT scan to rule out the presence of foreign body and perforating orbital injuries.
- Ask for thin orbital overlapping cuts with axial and coronal cuts in the CT scan (2 mm cuts).
- MRI should not be advised if metallic foreign body is suspected.

MANAGEMENT

- Reassurance.
- Ensure that the patient does not strain in any way.
- Shield the eye at the earliest.
- Nil per orally till advised, otherwise.
- Tetanus prophylaxis—tetanus toxoid/tetanus immunoglobulin.
- Inform the trauma consultant/duty consultant, anesthetist and operative theater staff.
- Urgent physician fitness/anesthetist fitness for GA to be obtained.
- Hospitalize the patient immediately.
- Prophylactic parenteral antibiotics (usually a combination of cefazolin and gentamycin)—tailored to the individual case.
- Surgery to be scheduled at the earliest.

SURGICAL MANAGEMENT (GENERAL GUIDELINES)

Anesthesia

- All open globe injuries to be repaired under GA.

- Peribulbar/parabulbar/retrobulbar anesthesia should be strictly avoided.
- If there is any life-threatening contraindication for GA, facial akinesia by O'Brien's/Van Lint technique can be combined with topical anesthesia.

Surgical Repair—Special Instructions

- Iris tissue when abscised to be sent for micro-biological examination.
- In case of retained intraocular foreign body with open globe VR surgeon to be informed urgently.
- Cases of open globe injury repaired elsewhere with retained intraocular foreign body to be seen by VR consultants.

CHEMICAL INJURIES

ETIOLOGY

Chemical injuries to the eye can result in mild injury, or severe ocular damage. Mostly victims are young and exposure occurs in workplace particularly in an industrial setting, at home, and in association with criminal assaults. Most chemical injuries are due to acid or alkali compounds, with the latter being more common.

The extent of ocular involvement depends on several factors:

- The strength of the chemical agent
- Concentration
- Volume of solution
- Duration of exposure.

PATHOPHYSIOLOGY

In general, alkalis tend to penetrate more effectively than acids.

Alkalis result in:

- Saponification and disruption of fatty acids in cell membranes, leading to cell death.
- Hydration of glycosaminoglycans results in loss of clarity of the stroma.
- Elevation in intraocular pressure.
- Intraocular structures may also be affected.
- Stromal corneal ulceration.

In acid injuries, the hydrogen ion causes damage due to pH alteration, while the anion produces protein precipitation and denaturation in the corneal epithelium and superficial stroma producing the ground glass appearance of the epithelium. This barrier may protect against weaker acids, but strong acids may continue to penetrate deeply.

CLASSIFICATION

A useful classification of chemical injuries was first proposed by Hughes and then modified by Roper-Hall (Table 8.1). This classification divides the clinical manifestations into four categories which help to guide prognosis and treatment. This classification has become the commonly used benchmark since its introduction in 1965.

Table 8.1: Classification of severity of ocular surface burns by Roper-Hall

Grade	Prognosis	Cornea	Conjunctiva / Limbus
I	Good	Corneal epithelial damage	No limbal ischemia
II	Good	Corneal haze, iris details visible	<1/3 limbal ischemia
III	Guarded	Total epithelial loss, stromal haze, iris details obscured	1/3–1/2 limbal ischemia
IV	Poor	Cornea opaque, iris and pupil obscured	>1/2 limbal ischemia

Dua et al proposed a significant modification to the Roper-Hall classification to take into account the extent of limbal involvement in clock hours, and the percentage of conjunctival involvement (Table 8.2). Clock hours of the limbus were determined by dividing the limbus into 12 hours of a clock face. It was concluded that with present management strategies like autolimbal or allolimbal transplantation, with or without amniotic membrane transplantation, an eye with 50 percent or even 75 percent limbal ischemia can expect a good to fair outcome, whereas an eye with 100 percent ischemia is very likely to have a poor outcome.

Table 8.2: New classification of ocular surface burns

Grade	Prognosis	Clinical findings	Conjunctival involvement	Analog scale*
I	Very good	O' clock hours of limbal involvement	0%	0/0%
II	Good	Up to 3 O' clock hours of limbal involvement	Up to 30%	0.1–3/ 1–29.9%
III	Good	>3–6 clock hours of limbal involvement	>30–50%	3.1–6/ 31–50%
IV	Good to guarded	>6–9 clock hours of limbal involvement	>50–75%	6.1–9/ 51–75%
V	Guarded to poor	>9–<12 clock hours of limbal involvement	>75–<100%	9.1–11.9/ 75.1–99.9%
VI	Very poor	Total limbus (12 O'clock hours) involved	Total conjunctiva (100%) involved	12/100%

* The analog scale records accurately the limbal involvement in clock hours of affected limbus/percentage of conjunctival involvement. While calculating percentage of conjunctival involvement, only involvement of bulbar conjunctiva, up to and including the conjunctival fornices is considered.

TREATMENT

Treatment can be divided into acute and chronic management strategies. Acute treatment is primarily medical, and chronic management may require surgical therapy. Management of chemical injury must attempt to:
1. Promote ocular surface epithelial recovery
2. Augment corneal repair
3. Control inflammation.

Treatment in the Acute Phase of Injury

Chemical injuries constitute a true ophthalmic emergency and immediate ocular irrigation is necessary prior to taking history, or completing the rest of the ocular examination.

- An isotonic solution with a neutral pH is preferable, such as normal saline or Ringer's lactate, any nontoxic solution is acceptable in an emergency. Irrigation should continue for a minimum of 30 minutes, or until the pH becomes neutral.
- Debridement of the necrotic corneal tissue.
- A broad-spectrum topical antibiotic such as ciprofloxacin would be prudent to avoid a microbial keratitis.
- Frequent lubrication with preservative free eye drops should be utilized to enhance epithelialization.
- Bandage soft contact lenses with careful follow-up.
- Topical corticosteroids can be utilized to decrease inflammation in the first 7 to 10 days of treatment.
- Topical NSAIDs such as ketoralac.
- Sodium ascorbate 10 percent hourly or 1000 mg of oral ascorbic acid four times.
- Tetracycline and its derivatives may be added for anticollagenolytic effect.
- Sodium citrate 10 percent hourly.
- A glass rod can be used to break developing symblepharon on a daily basis and helps to prevent shortening of fornices. Alternatively a symblepharon ring can be used with a bandage contact lens.
- Tissue adhesives like cyanoacrylate glue are effective tool for management of impending or actual perforation related to sterile ulceration of the corneal stroma following chemical injury.

Surgical Management in Acute Phase

- *Amniotic membrane transplant (AMT):* For large non-healing epithelial defects, amniotic membrane transplantation can be performed in the acute stage.
- *Tenonplasty:* It is recommended in cases of persistent scleral and limbal ischemia in combination with amniotic membrane transplantation.

- *Tectonic graft:* It is performed in case of large corneal perforation.

Management in Chronic Phase

Prior to undertaking any visual rehabilitative procedures, it is extremely important to correct any associated glaucoma through medical and/or surgical means and address surface inflammation. Fornix reconstruction forms the initial phase of rehabilitation in order to stabilize the tear film and better the success of subsequent limbal transplantation.

Limbal Stem Cell Transplantation

In unilateral chemical injuries with total limbal stem cell deficiency, the procedure of choice would conjunctival limbal autograft (CLAU).

It is usually performed in a staged manner:
- Fornix reconstruction.
- Limbal autograft (CLAU or *ex-vivo* limbal stem cell transplant).
- Lamellar or penetrating keratoplasty for corneal opacity.

In bilateral chemical injuries, limbal allograft can be performed. However, this procedure is associated with a high risk of rejection and requires long-term immunosuppression.

Keratoprosthesis may be useful for bilateral, severe chemical injury where the prognosis is hopeless for penetrating keratoplasty due to irreparable damage to the ocular surface or repeated immunological rejection.

- Boston KPro has established its role in restoring vision to patients suffering from corneal blindness from various pathologies including chemical injuries. Overall, the Boston KPro is capable of restoring media clarity and demonstrates good anatomic retention. But patients with chemical burns are more difficult group to manage due to presence of concomitant preoperative ocular disease, particularly glaucoma and high extrusion rates.

- Modified osteo-odonto-keratoprosthesis that uses the autologous tooth as a carrier for the polymethyl-methacrylate is reserved for the more severe cases of chemical injury. It has shown to provide long-term, anatomically stable corneal prosthesis as well as an effective rehabilitating recovery in visual acuity.

CLOSED GLOBE INJURIES

- Traumatic hyphema
- Traumatic uveitis
- Lens injuries
- Angle recession and glaucoma
- Traumatic optic neuropathy
- Posterior segment and retinal dialysis
- Giant retinal tear.

HYPHEMA

History

- Mechanism (force and direction).
- Size of the object (e.g. shuttle cock causes more damage than tennis ball).
- Time of injury.

Examination

- Check pinhole visual acuity.
- Pupillary examination for RAPD.
- *Slit-lamp examination:*
  - Suspect globe rupture in eyes with dense subconjunctival hemorrhage, subconjunctival pigment or soft eye.
  - Corneal status-corneal edema/staining, etc.
  - Level of hyphema.
  - Other anterior segment injuries if any, e.g. lens subluxation iridodialysis, etc.
  - Check IOP with applanation tonometry or tonopen (if cornea is edematous).
- Defer gonioscopy. Use Zeiss gonioscopy if necessary.
- Fundus examination by indirect ophthalmoscopy. Avoid scleral depression.

Investigations

- Ultrasound examination

- Posterior segment status
- Occult globe rupture
- Optic nerve injuries
- Orbital hemorrhage.
- *Ultrasound biomicroscopy (UBM):* To evaluate the anterior segment details like, zonular dialysis, ciliochoroidal detachment, etc. where appropriate.
- CT scan if orbital injuries are suspected.
- Visual evoked potential (VEP) to be done when RAPD is noted and clinical evidence suggests optic nerve injury.

Management

Factors which influence the treatment are:
- The level of hyphema and IOP
- Corneal blood staining
- Duration of hyphema.

Medical Management

- If the hyphema is <1/2 without corneal staining, IOP < 30 mm Hg, management is conservative.
- Advise strict bed rest.
- Protective eye shield to prevent further trauma.
- Topical steroids and cycloplegic.
- *Antiglaucoma medications:*
    - Start β-blockers.
    - Oral acetazolamide as a routine until otherwise contraindicated (IV mannitol to be used If the IOP is very high and not responding to topical β-blockers and oral acetazolamide).
- *Hospitalize the patient:*
    - If there is total hyphema and IOP is very high (e.g. more than 50 mm Hg even after the use of IV mannitol).
    - Poor compliance of the patient.
    - Pediatric cases where the treatment may not be possible at home.

Surgical Management

- *Anterior chamber evacuation done in cases of:*
  - Total hyphema with corneal staining.
  - Increased IOP not responding to antiglaucoma medications (e.g. 30 mm Hg × 7 days or 50 mm Hg × 5 day).

Follow-up

- Frequent follow-up during the first few weeks of injury.
- *During every follow-up visit:*
  - Visual acuity
  - Look for rebleed
  - Monitor intraocular pressure
  - Anterior chamber reaction.
- Treatment to be adjusted accordingly.
- Gonioscopy to rule out angle recession.
- Fundus examination by indirect ophthalmoscopy with depression to be done as a routine 2 weeks post-trauma.

TRAUMATIC UVEITIS

- Must be looked for carefully in all cases.
- Check for anterior chamber cells and flare using proper technique, i.e. darkroom, etc.
- Treat with topical steroids, cycloplegics; oral steroids in severe cases.

LENS INJURIES

- History is same as mentioned for hyphema.
- *Complete examination:*
  - Look for subluxation/dislocation and degree of zonular dialysis in all blunt trauma patients.
  - Look for other associated anterior segment injuries.
  - Gonioscopy, indirect ophthalmoscopy with depression to be done two weeks after the injury.

- Consider UBM to evaluate the degree of zonular dialysis, so that surgical management can be planned accordingly.
- If there is any associated uveitis, to be treated with topical steroids and cycloplegics.
- Plan for early surgical intervention if there is a disruption of the capsule.

TRAUMATIC ANGLE RECESSION/GLAUCOMA

- It is not a separate entity and usually presents along with other features of blunt trauma.
- Careful angle study in all cases of blunt trauma two weeks after the injury as mentioned earlier. Always compare the angle of normal eye.
- Check IOP at frequent intervals during 1st few weeks after injury.
- Explain the possibility of glaucoma in all patients with angle recession and need for regular follow-up.

COMMOTIO RETINAE (BERLIN'S EDEMA)

Examination

Complete eye examination including fundus examination with dilated pupils as early as possible:
- Look carefully at the disc and entire retina.
- Commotio retinae results in retinal whitening and is most commonly seen in the posterior pole (Berlin's edema).

Management

The condition clears in 3 to 4 weeks, and prognosis for visual recovery is good.
- There is no treatment.
- Oral steroids may be prescribed based on severity, and associated inflammation.

TRAUMATIC OPTIC NEUROPATHY

It is optic neuropathy that is temporally related to blunt or penetrating head trauma that results following road traffic accidents, fall from a height or from frontal impact by falling debris, assault, stab wounds and gunshot wounds. May result following iatrogenic injury such as endoscopic sinus surgery or orbital surgery. Rarely results from orbital hemorrhage (retrobulbar hemorrhage) or orbital emphysema.

They are divided into:
- Direct injury that results from orbital or cerebral trauma that transgresses normal tissue planes to disrupt the anatomic and functional integrity of the optic nerve, e.g. bullet penetrating orbit. Vision loss is severe, immediate and recovery is unlikely.
- Indirect injury usually results from blunt trauma to the forehead that results in transmission of force through the cranium to the restrained intra-canalicular portion of optic nerve. Vision loss may be delayed and recovery is poor.

They are classified into three types:
- Optic nerve avulsion—ophthalmoscopic appearance consists of a partial ring of hemorrhage or the avulsion can be seen as a dark crescentic area.
- Anterior optic neuropathy—injury within 10 mm of the globe. Central retinal artery occlusion or vein occlusion may occur.
- Posterior optic neuropathy—injury posterior to entrance of central retinal artery or vein.

Clinical Features
- Vision varies from no perception of light to 6/6. Associated field defect is present—altitudinal, central, paracentral, centrocecal. Injury to intracranial optic

nerve produces hemianopic field defect. Relative afferent pupillary defect is present in unilateral injury. Multisystem trauma or serious brain damage with loss of consciousness may be present.

- In some cases no evidence of orbital or ocular trauma is seen. Others may have periorbital or ocular hemorrhage, ecchymosis or laceration.

Investigations

- Visual evoked potential—helps in assessing optic nerve function in an unresponsive patient.
- CT scan orbit and brain—look for optic canal fracture fragments which can be impinging on the nerve.
- MRI—helps in evaluating intracranial abnormalities, can detect subtle hemorrhage of the optic nerve or its sheath.

Management

- Respiratory and cardiovascular resuscitation and stabilization are the first priority. Care of the patient may need a team approach. Treatment is based on the United States National Acute Spinal Cord Injury Study. Within eight hours of injury patients should receive intravenous methylprednisolone at the rate of 30 mg/kg loading dose followed by a continuous infusion of 5.4 mg/kg/hour for 48 hours.
- If vision does not improve in 48 hours, optic nerve decompression may be considered. Cases with bony fragments impinging on the optic nerve will need decompression and evacuation of optic nerve sheath hematoma.
- Some cases can improve on their own without treatment.

EYELID AND ADNEXAL INJURIES

HISTORY

- Details of injury.
- Possibility of FB.
- First aid, details of treatment taken earlier including injury tetanus toxoid.
- Any associated injuries—head injuries, fractures.
- General condition—systemic disease.

EXAMINATION

- Use disposable gloves.
- Evaluate the general condition.
  - If sick or unstable, urgent evaluation by physician/anesthetist/consultant in the emergency.
  - Immediately transfer the patient to an appropriate hospital.
- All injuries to be examined and described in detail—a simple diagrammatic representation is appropriate.
- Remove any glass pieces, dirt or foreign material.
- Clean wound with saline/distilled water.
- Evaluate pupils—RAPD.
- In case of profuse bleeding, inform the oculoplasty/trauma consultant urgently.
- Look for associated orbital injuries—hematoma, fractures.
- Perform a complete ophthalmic examination in all cases and rule out associated globe injuries.
- Partial thickness/full thickness injury.
- Injury involving lid margin or sparing.
- Condition of punctum and canaliculus to be assessed.

MANAGEMENT

- *In emergency department:*
  - Documentation of injuries if possible.
  - Injury TT 0.5 ml IM (if not already given).
  - Nil orally till further orders.
  - Physician/anesthetist opinion for fitness as appropriate.
  - Oculoplasty/trauma consultant to be informed urgently.
  - Arrange repair/reconstruction.
- *In operation theater:*
  - Complete documentation of injuries under anesthesia.
  - Urgent repair/reconstruction of eyelid injuries.
  - Evaluate eye-globe repair if perforating injuries are present.
  - If no associated globe injuries, lid surgery to be scheduled within 24 hours.
  - Repair may necessitate specialized techniques, e.g. skin grafting in injuries with loss of tissue, eyelid burns.
- Postoperative evaluation at regular intervals.

ORBITAL INJURIES INCLUDING FRACTURES

HISTORY

- Details of mode of injury—exact detailed description to be obtained from patient, witnesses.
- Possibility of FBs to be explored by detailed history.
- First aid, details of treatment taken earlier including Injury tetanus toxoid.
- Any associated injuries—head injuries, fractures, etc. to be specifically asked for.
- General condition—systemic disease.
- History of double vision, numbness or abnormal sensations over lower lid, cheek, or upper lid of affected side to be asked for.
- Difficulty in opening mouth, chewing, etc.

EXAMINATION

- Use disposable gloves when examining the patient.
- Evaluate the general condition of the patient and if sick or unstable, urgent evaluation by physician/ anesthetist/consultant in the emergency.
- If general condition is poor, a decision regarding shifting the patient out of Sankara Nethralaya and to an appropriate hospital may need to be taken urgently.
- All injuries to be examined and described in detail; a simple diagrammatic representation is appropriate.
- Rule out globe injury.
- Remove any glass pieces, dirt or foreign material and clean the wound with saline/distilled water.
- In case of profuse bleeding, inform the oculoplasty/ trauma consultant urgently.
- Evaluate pupils and rule out RAPD in all cases.
- In case of profuse bleeding, inform the oculoplasty/ trauma consultant urgently.

- Look for and rule out proptosis/enophthalmos.
- Rule out subcutaneous emphysema by looking for crepitus.
- Gently palpate the orbital margins and facial bones for any point tenderness, irregularity or deformity.
- Evaluate ocular motility and look for double vision.
- Document double vision with Hess and diplopia charting whenever possible.
- Perform Hertel's exophthalmometry whenever required and possible.
- Rule out infraorbital nerve hypoesthesia.

MANAGEMENT

- Photographic documentation of all cases.
- In case of proptosis, lubricant therapy, taping as applicable to prevent corneal exposure.
- Ultrasound examination of orbit to rule out hematoma, etc. when needed.
- X-ray orbits, CT scan orbit with axial and coronal cuts for documentation and to rule out fractures.
- Oral antibiotics, NSAIDs, etc. as appropriate.
- Use of ice packs in the early stages post injury to reduce swelling, pain.
- Injection TT 0.5 ml intramuscular if not already given.
- Inform trauma/oculoplasty consultant.
- Advise patient not to blow the nose, especially if fracture of the medial orbital wall is suspected.
- Conservative/surgical treatment on basis of extent of fractures, symptoms and signs. Surgical repair usually after 10 to 14 days .
- Serial Hess and diplopia charting to evaluate progress.
- Referral to faciomaxillary surgeon or neurosurgeon when appropriate.

GUIDELINES FOR THE EMERGENCY DOCTORS

- Patients with eye conditions which need urgent attention are seen in the emergency department manned by emergency doctors (Postgraduates and fellows). This service is provided round the clock. Treatment of minor eye ailments is done by the emergency doctors, if needed, after consultation with the concerned consultant.
- Patients needing more specialized care including surgical treatment are seen by the concerned consultant (trauma, vitreoretinal, cornea, glaucoma, etc.) during routine working hours (8 am–5 pm) and by the duty consultant in the afterhours who advises regarding treatment, if needed, after consultation with the concerned consultant, and undertakes emergency operations, e.g. repair of open globe injuries. The duty consultant is on call and is informed regarding the patients seen in the emergency.

INDEX